NEUROLOGY – LABORATORY AND
CLINICAL RESEARCH DEVELOPMENTS

UNDERSTANDING DYSKINESIA

NEUROLOGY – LABORATORY AND CLINICAL RESEARCH DEVELOPMENTS

Additional books and e-books in this series can be found on Nova's website under the Series tab.

NEUROLOGY – LABORATORY AND
CLINICAL RESEARCH DEVELOPMENTS

UNDERSTANDING DYSKINESIA

JAN DVOŘÁK
EDITOR

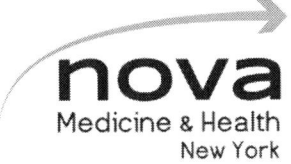

Copyright © 2020 by Nova Science Publishers, Inc.

All rights reserved. No part of this book may be reproduced, stored in a retrieval system or transmitted in any form or by any means: electronic, electrostatic, magnetic, tape, mechanical photocopying, recording or otherwise without the written permission of the Publisher.

We have partnered with Copyright Clearance Center to make it easy for you to obtain permissions to reuse content from this publication. Simply navigate to this publication's page on Nova's website and locate the "Get Permission" button below the title description. This button is linked directly to the title's permission page on copyright.com. Alternatively, you can visit copyright.com and search by title, ISBN, or ISSN.

For further questions about using the service on copyright.com, please contact:
Copyright Clearance Center
Phone: +1-(978) 750-8400   Fax: +1-(978) 750-4470   E-mail: info@copyright.com

NOTICE TO THE READER

The Publisher has taken reasonable care in the preparation of this book, but makes no expressed or implied warranty of any kind and assumes no responsibility for any errors or omissions. No liability is assumed for incidental or consequential damages in connection with or arising out of information contained in this book. The Publisher shall not be liable for any special, consequential, or exemplary damages resulting, in whole or in part, from the readers' use of, or reliance upon, this material. Any parts of this book based on government reports are so indicated and copyright is claimed for those parts to the extent applicable to compilations of such works.

Independent verification should be sought for any data, advice or recommendations contained in this book. In addition, no responsibility is assumed by the Publisher for any injury and/or damage to persons or property arising from any methods, products, instructions, ideas or otherwise contained in this publication.

This publication is designed to provide accurate and authoritative information with regard to the subject matter covered herein. It is sold with the clear understanding that the Publisher is not engaged in rendering legal or any other professional services. If legal or any other expert assistance is required, the services of a competent person should be sought. FROM A DECLARATION OF PARTICIPANTS JOINTLY ADOPTED BY A COMMITTEE OF THE AMERICAN BAR ASSOCIATION AND A COMMITTEE OF PUBLISHERS.

Additional color graphics may be available in the e-book version of this book.

Library of Congress Cataloging-in-Publication Data

Names: Dvořák, Jan (Nova Publishers editor) editor.
Title: Understanding dyskinesia / Jan Dvořák, editor.
Description: New York : Nova Science Publishers, [2020] | Series: Neurology
  - laboratory and clinical research developments | Includes
  bibliographical references and index. |
Identifiers: LCCN 2020037155 (print) | LCCN 2020037156 (ebook) | ISBN
  9781536185027 (hardcover) | ISBN 9781536184907 (adobe pdf)
Subjects: LCSH: Tardive dyskinesia.
Classification: LCC RC394.T37 U53 2020 (print) | LCC RC394.T37 (ebook) |
  DDC 616.8/3--dc23
LC record available at https://lccn.loc.gov/2020037155
LC ebook record available at https://lccn.loc.gov/2020037156

Published by Nova Science Publishers, Inc. † New York

Contents

Preface		vii
Chapter 1	Primary Ciliary Dyskinesia *Ana Reula, Antonio Moreno-Galdó, Sandra Rovira-Amigó, Núria Camats-Tarruella, Teresa Jaijo, Noelia Baz-Redón, Carmen Carda, Lara Milian, Manuel Mata and Miguel Armengot-Carceller*	1
Chapter 2	Tardive Dyskinesia and Mental Illness: A Systematic Review *Alfonso Pedrós Roselló, Francesc Pascual Sanchis, Raquel Úbeda Cano, Begoña Pérez Longás, Dimitri Malventi Bellido and Teresa Pedrós Diago*	69
Chapter 3	Physical Activity, Exercise and Dyskinesia *Ana Elisa Speck, Rui Daniel Schroder Prediger and Aderbal Silva Aguiar Junior*	103
Bibliography		131
Related Nova Publications		179
Index		185

Preface

Primary Ciliary Dyskinesia is a rare disease with a prevalence of 1:20.000 births (ORPHA244). Understanding Dyskinesia aims to give an overview of what primary ciliary dyskinesia is, the differences in patients' clinical manifestations throughout their lives, its genetics, and diagnostic tests available for this disease.

The authors present a systematic review of tardive dyskinesia, covering the clinical manifestations, epidemiology, etiology, and an update on the therapeutic approach.

In addition, the acute effects of physical activity and exercise adaptation on different types of dyskinesia are assessed.

Chapter 1 - Primary Ciliary Dyskinesia (PCD) is a rare disease with a prevalence of 1:20.000 births (ORPHA244). It is a genetic disease characterised by abnormal motility or immotility of motile cilia and flagella. Thus, PCD patients have impaired mucociliary clearance of secretions, bacteria, pollutants, and allergens from upper and lower airways. PCD is related to fertility issues because Fallopian tubes' cilia and spermatozoa are affected. Moreover, a random distribution of the organs because of embryonic nodal cilia affectation produces situs inversus in 50% of the cases and situs ambiguous in 6%.

PCD is a heterogeneous disease, which comprises symptoms that could be confused with other diseases like Cystic Fibrosis. Clinical manifestations often start from birth and are persistent throughout life. Despite being a genetic disease with an autosomal recessive inheritance in the majority of the cases, PCD is a genetically heterogeneous disease. To date, mutations in more than 40 genes have been identified, and these only explain 65% of PCD cases.

There is no gold standard diagnostic test for PCD, so a combination of diagnostic tests is required: ciliary beat frequency and pattern analysis by High Speed Video Microscopy (HSVM), ciliary ultrastructure study by Transmission Electron Microscopy (TEM), and genetic testing. Moreover, nasal Nitric Oxide (nNO) levels are used as a screening test, and immunofluorescence staining of specific ciliary structure proteins is becoming a potential diagnostic test that is yet to be validated. Despite having therapeutic options that contribute to wellbeing, to date, there is no specific treatment for PCD patients.

This chapter aims to give an overview of what PCD is, the differences in patients' clinical manifestations throughout their life, its genetics, and diagnostic tests available for this disease.

Chapter 2 - Tardive dyskinesia (TD) remains as an important clinical problem, causing severe limitations in daily life. It is a hyperkinetic movement disorder caused by the prolonged use of neuroleptics (NL), with a prevalence of 20-25%. It is classified as an extrapyramidal side effect induced by these drugs. Due to its severity, a proper assessment and monitoring of patients is necessary in order to avoid or reduce its intensity. However, with the emergence of new neuroleptics, new paths of hope have appeared, as the extrapyramidal profile of these molecules is more favorable than that of classical neuroleptics. The best way to minimize the risk of developing TD is to prevent it. This preventive approach should always be taken into account in patients with mental illness.

This chapter presents a systematic review of TD, covering the clinical manifestations, epidemiology, etiology, and an update on the therapeutic approach.

Chapter 3 - Dyskinesia is hyperkinetic abnormal involuntary movement (AIM) which includes isolated or combined chorea, dystonia, athetosis, and ballism. AIM can be found in some disorders, such as Levodopa-induced dyskinesia (LIDs) in Parkinson's disease, tardive dyskinesia in schizophrenia, and paroxysmal dyskinesia. The purpose of this chapter is to review the acute effects of physical activity and exercise adaptation (eg rehabilitation) on different types of dyskinesia. Physical activity showed antidyskinetic effects in Parkinson's LIDs, with well-defined biological mechanisms. Acute exercise does not modify abnormal respiratory patters in schizophrenia. These patients have a normal response to progressive exercise and inspiratory time. Sustained walking or running may induce paroxysmal dyskinesia in healthy subjects. The authors will deeply explore this evidence.

In: Understanding Dyskinesia
Editor: Jan Dvořák
ISBN: 978-1-53618-502-7
© 2020 Nova Science Publishers, Inc.

Chapter 1

PRIMARY CILIARY DYSKINESIA

Ana Reula[1,2,], PhD, Antonio Moreno-Galdó[3,4,5,6], PhD,*
Sandra Rovira-Amigó[3,4,5], MD,
Núria Camats-Tarruella[3,6], PhD, Teresa Jaijo[2,6,7], PhD,
Noelia Baz-Redón[3,4], Carmen Carda[1], PhD,
Lara Milian[1], PhD, Manuel Mata[1,8], PhD
and Miguel Armengot-Carceller [2,9,10,11], PhD

[1]Pathology Department, University of Valencia, Valencia, Spain
[2]Molecular, Cellular and Genomic Biomedicine Group, IIS La Fe, Valencia, Spain
[3]Vall d'Hebron Research Institute, Hospital Universitario Vall d'Hebron, Barcelona, Spain
[4]Paediatrics, Obstetrics and Gynaecology Department, Universitat Autònoma de Barcelona, Barcelona, Spain
[5]Paediatrics Allergology, Pneumology and Cystic Fibrosis Section, Hospital Universitari Vall d'Hebron, Barcelona, Spain
[6]CIBERER, Instituto de Salud Carlos III, ISCIII), Madrid, Spain

---

[*] Corresponding Author's Email: ana.reula@uv.es.

[7]Genetics and Prenatal Diagnostic Unit, Hospital Universitario y Politécnico La Fe, Valencia, Spain
[8]Research Institute of the University Clinical Hospital of Valencia (INCLIVA), Valencia, Spain
[9]CIBERES, Instituto de Salud Carlos III (ISCIII), Madrid, Spain
[10]Surgery Department. University of Valencia, Valencia, Spain
[11]ENT Service, Hospital Universitario y Politécnico La Fe, Valencia, Spain

ABSTRACT

Primary Ciliary Dyskinesia (PCD) is a rare disease with a prevalence of 1:20.000 births (ORPHA244). It is a genetic disease characterised by abnormal motility or immotility of motile cilia and flagella. Thus, PCD patients have impaired mucociliary clearance of secretions, bacteria, pollutants, and allergens from upper and lower airways. PCD is related to fertility issues because Fallopian tubes' cilia and spermatozoa are affected. Moreover, a random distribution of the organs because of embryonic nodal cilia affectation produces situs inversus in 50% of the cases and situs ambiguous in 6% [1].

PCD is a heterogeneous disease, which comprises symptoms that could be confused with other diseases like Cystic Fibrosis. Clinical manifestations often start from birth and are persistent throughout life. Despite being a genetic disease with an autosomal recessive inheritance in the majority of the cases, PCD is a genetically heterogeneous disease. To date, mutations in more than 40 genes have been identified, and these only explain 65% of PCD cases [2].

There is no gold standard diagnostic test for PCD, so a combination of diagnostic tests is required: ciliary beat frequency and pattern analysis by High Speed Video Microscopy (HSVM), ciliary ultrastructure study by Transmission Electron Microscopy (TEM), and genetic testing [3]. Moreover, nasal Nitric Oxide (nNO) levels are used as a screening test [2], and immunofluorescence staining of specific ciliary structure proteins is becoming a potential diagnostic test that is yet to be validated [4]. Despite having therapeutic options that contribute to wellbeing, to date, there is no specific treatment for PCD patients [5].

This chapter aims to give an overview of what PCD is, the differences in patients' clinical manifestations throughout their life, its genetics, and diagnostic tests available for this disease.

1. INTRODUCTION

1.1. Cilia Structure and Function

Cilia are cellular organelles that have been conserved by evolution. They are present in many unicellular and some cells of multicellular organisms. They are classified as primary or sensitive cilia and motile ones. First ones, immotile, are information sensors which are present in sight, hearing and smell organs, renal tubular epithelial cells, and in most body cells at some point in evolution. The second ones are located in the epithelial surface of the respiratory tract, ependymal tissue, and reproductive male and female organs (testicular efferent and Fallopian tubes). Also, sperm tail has a ciliary structure modified to flagellum [6].

Cilia are cell projections covered by a cell membrane, which have a motoric function that direct particles propulsion through a fluid, or liquid, on the cell surface. The main structure is called axonema, which in motile cilia has a characteristic 9+2 organization: a central pair of internal microtubules, surrounded by 9 peripheral microtubules' doublets (Figure 1). Peripheral microtubules are joined between them by nexin links, and to the central pair by radial spokes. Dynein complexes are associated with peripheral microtubules, represented as external and internal dynein arms of doublets [7].

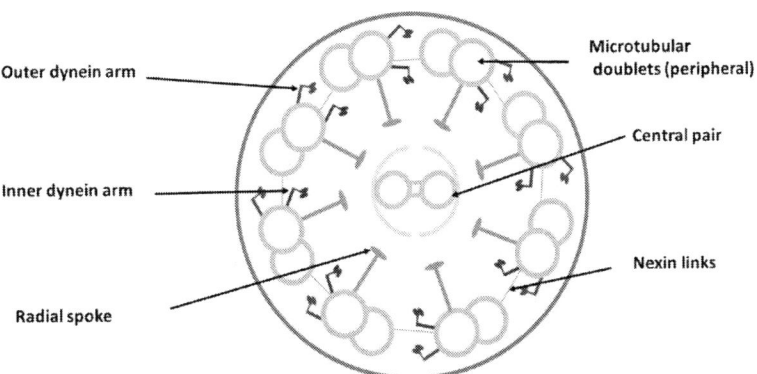

Figure 1. Transversal section of cilia axoneme indicating ultrastructural parts.

Dynein arms are connected with ATPases that generate movement by ATP hydrolysis. Thus, dynein is directly related to motoric cilia function, and radial spokes determine movement direction [8].

1.2. Disease History

In 1901, the association between situs inversus and bronchiectasis was for the first time described by Siewert [9]. After that, in 1933, Kartagener studied a group of patients with bronchiectasis, situs inversus and sinusitis [10]. Since that moment, this symptoms' triad was known as Kartagener syndrome.

In 1975, Afzelius identified structural abnormalities in sperms of an infertile men group, that also presented chronic bronchitis and bronchiectasis [11]. Subsequent studies detected similar alterations in respiratory tract cilia [12]. Two years later, various clinical cases compatible with "Kartagener syndrome", with the same ultrastructural abnormalities but without situs inversus were published [13]. This is why in 1980, "immotile cilia syndrome" was proposed in reference to these cases, as situs inversus was only present in around 50% of cases [14, 15], leaving "Kartagener syndrome" term for those patients presenting the complete triad of symptoms.

Later, in 1988, it was demonstrated that clinical manifestations were not only due to immotile cilia, but also due to dyskinetic or inefficient cilia movement. Thus, "Primary Ciliary Dyskinesia" substituted "immotile cilia syndrome" term [16].

In the late 80s, it was demonstrated that mucociliary transport could be altered, not only due to ultrastructural cilia defects, but also due to bacterial or viral recurrent infections or by inhalation of substances or drugs that by altering ciliary function, cause stasis of secretions, reproducing a PCD clinical picture [17]. At the same time, recurrent infections could lead to a chronic inflammatory process in airways that could affect cilia ultrastructure [18]. So "Secondary Ciliary Dyskinesia" term was defined to refer to transitory alterations in mucociliary transport due to secondary causes, while PCD was referred to an hereditary and permanent condition [19].

1.3. Primary Ciliary Dyskinesia in Rare Diseases Context

Rare Diseases are those that affect a small number of patients inside the general population. In Europe, a disease is considered rare when it affects 1 individual in 2.000 [20]. According to World Health Organization, there are about 8.000 rare diseases, and although each of them affects a small number of people, the total number of patients with these diseases is 7% of the world's population (over 400 million). PCD (ORPHA244) is the second most common congenital affection that affects respiratory tract after Cystic Fibrosis, with an estimated prevalence of 1/20.000, so it can be considered a rare disease [20].

It is an underdiagnosed disease with an obvious diagnostic delay, although the symptoms appear at a very early age. In Europe, the average age at diagnosis is 5.3 years, and it reduces to 3.5 years in patients who present situs inversus [21]. Khueni et al. appreciate that there is a correlation between early diagnosis and greater government investment in health. They found out that while the average diagnostic age in the British Isles is 4.8 years, in Western and Northern Europe and Eastern and Southern Europe, it is 5 and 5.5 and 6.8 and 6.5 years, respectively [22].

This study, carried out by the European Respiratory Society Task Force, in which a total of 223 centers from 26 European countries participated and more than 1.000 patients diagnosed with PCD before the age of 20 were collected, concludes that the prevalence of the disease is very variable between different countries. Thus, in Cyprus there was the highest frequency (111 cases per million inhabitants between 5-14 years, which is equivalent to 1/10.000); Denmark or Switzerland had a prevalence of 1/20.000, and Spain of 20.5 cases per million inhabitants (1/30.000 children) [22].

2. Clinical Manifestations in Children

Diagnosis of PCD is frequently delayed, in part because patients present symptoms (rhinitis, secretory otitis media, cough, and recurrent bronchitis) that are common in children [5]. Symptoms start very early in life and even some antenatal manifestations can be present [1].

Approximately 40–55% of the affected children have situs inversus [22, 23]. It is estimated that 25% of people with situs inversus have PCD [24]. About 6-12% with PCD have heterotaxy (situs ambiguous), frequently associated with intracardiac defect [25, 26]. Radial spoke, central pair and isolated nexin link defects do not present with laterality defects because they are not present in embryonic nodal cilia, as well as genes associated with reduced generation of motile cilia (*MCIDAS, CCNO*).

Mild cerebral ventriculomegaly, sometimes transient, could be an early sign of PCD [27]. One of 40 individuals with PCD shows hydrocephalus, which is present in 10% of patients with *CCNO* mutations [28].

PCD often (75-85%) presents at birth with unexplained neonatal respiratory distress [1, 29, 30]. Infants develop respiratory distress after a few hours of life (12-24 h) and often need supplemental oxygen for several days [23]. Lobar collapse of the upper and middle lobe is a frequent complication in the neonatal period.

Upper and lower respiratory tract symptoms and recurrent and chronic respiratory infections start soon after birth.

Chronic nasal congestion and chronic daily wet cough start at a median of 1 month of age. Cough frequency is greater during the day than at night. It can partially improve with antibiotic therapy but does not resolve with therapy or changes of season [23, 24, 31].

Chronic or recurrent otitis media with effusion is very common and is often associated with conductive hearing difficulty. Persistent otorrhea can occur after ventilation tube insertion. Symptoms of sinusitis often develop in childhood. Nasal polyposis is rare in children [32, 33].

Recurrent pulmonary infections lead to bronchiectasis that is present in 50-60% of children. They typically occur in the middle and lower lobes, which can be a distinguishing feature from cystic fibrosis (CF) [34, 35].

The most common respiratory pathogens in children are *Haemophilus influenzae, Streptococcus pneumoniae, Staphylococcus aureus* and *Moraxella catarrhalis. Pseudomonas aeruginosa* may appear but it is more prevalent in adults [36, 37].

A systematic review and meta-analysis included 52 studies with 1970 paediatrics and adults' patients. They found a prevalence of 5% for congenital heart disease in PCD patients. There was a considerable heterogeneity between-studies in symptoms' prevalence. The mean prevalence of situs anomalies was 49%, chronic cough 89%, lower respiratory tract infections 72%, chronic rhinitis 75%, bronchiectasis 56%, otitis media 74%, hypoacusia 36%, and nasal polyps 19% [38].

There is some influence of genotype on clinical presentation. Some genes affecting motile cilia are associated with more severe diseases like *CCD39* and *CCDC40* [39], while others are associated with milder diseases because some mucociliary clearance is maintained (*DNAH9*) [40]. Even some newly described (*MNS1* [41], *ENKUR* [42]) genes cause situs inversus without significant chest disease. Patients with reduced numbers of motile cilia (*CCNO* and *MCIDAS*) have a severe respiratory phenotype with a rapid deterioration of lung function [28].

3. CLINICAL MANIFESTATIONS IN ADULTS

Clinical manifestations, which begin in newborns, persist perennially throughout life. The patients' quality of life, however, worsens over the years. This worsening or aggravation is due to different factors, not only physical but also social, emotional, and the negative impact of treatment itself [43]. It is also necessary to consider that this disease affects the growth and development of patients. A longitudinal study over time [44] analyzes the evolution of height, weight and body mass index (BMI) of patients with PCD, concluding that in these patients, there is a serious deterioration of growth during childhood, up to 17 years. In addition, such deterioration is not related to sex or severity of the disease but was more pronounced in *DNAH5* or *DNAI1* mutation carriers

Daily wet cough, chronic rhinorrhea, and hypoacusia persist throughout adulthood. All this symptomatology shows a poor response to treatments that are established in patients with the same clinic but do not suffer from PCD. Studies that analyze both clinical manifestations and treatment are scarcer when they refer to adults than children [45]. Starting from the common symptomatology, which always exists, this disease can progress to greater severity in some patients. [23].

In this section, we highlight the most specific aspects of both clinical manifestations and treatment in adults.

3.1. ENT Clinical Manifestations

Perennial mucopurulent rhinitis responds poorly to standard treatments and is often complicated by sinusitis in older children and adults. Hearing loss is also a common symptom in adult patients with PCD, it is usually permanent, although with typical secretory otitis media fluctuations [1].

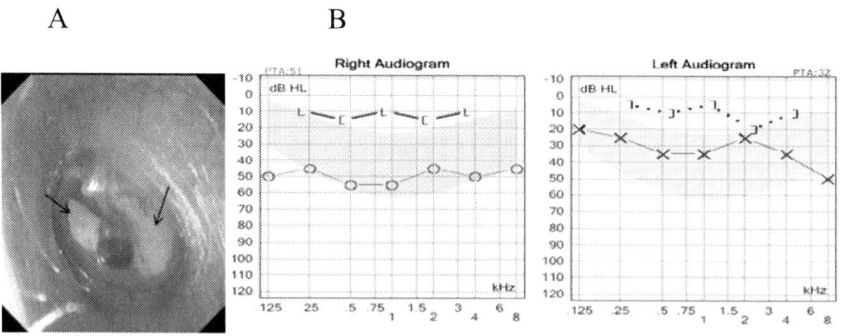

Figure 2. Ear problems in PCD. A) Seromucous chronic otitis media and tympanosclerosis (arrows). B) Transmission hearing loss.

Ear problems generally improve with age, but patients may have permanent conductive hearing loss [46]. Secretory otitis media is a common finding in adult patients, although its presence and severity are less in children (Figure 2). However, in a third of PCD adults, a sensorineural hearing loss, probably as a consequence of otitis media chronicity, is detected. Secondary to the long evolution of secretory otitis and frequent superinfections, it is common to find tympanosclerosis plaques in the eardrum [47]).

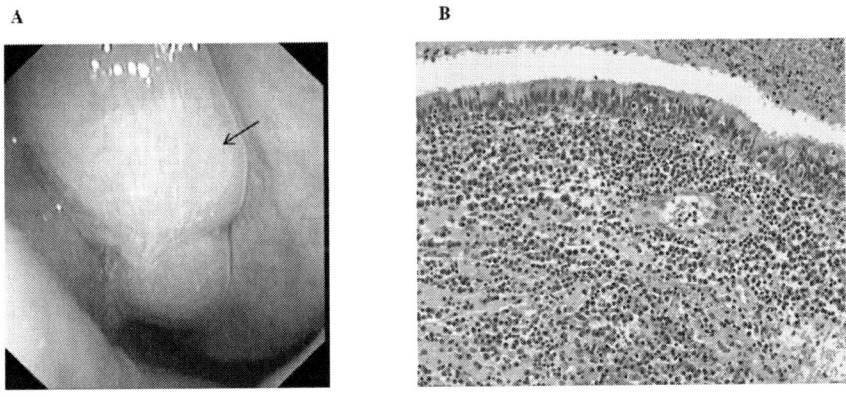

Figure 3. Nasal polyps in PCD. A) Fibrous looking polyps (arrow). B) Neutrophilic polyposis.

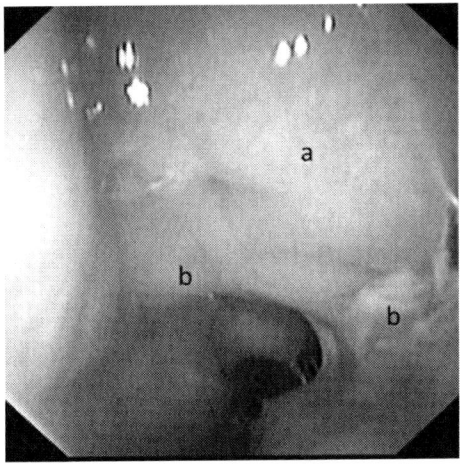

Figure 4. Nasal endoscopy in PCD: Mucosal congestion (a) and rhinorrea in nasal meatus (b).

Chronic rhinosinusitis is the most common clinical feature of PCD in adults. Nasal polyposis is less common than in CF, affecting 15-30% of patients [30, 47], but these polyps are neutrophilic and fibromatous (Figure 3), unlike what happens in idiopathic polyposis, where the polyps are edematous and eosinophilic. Congestive nasal mucous membranes and mucopurulent secretion in all nasal meatus is common in all adult patients (Figure 4). PCD patients often have hypoplasia of paranasal sinuses, and especially, frontal sinus aplasia evidenced when performing a computed tomography scan (CT). A partial or total occupation of all sinuses is also common, which is known as pansinusitis (Figure 5) [1, 47].

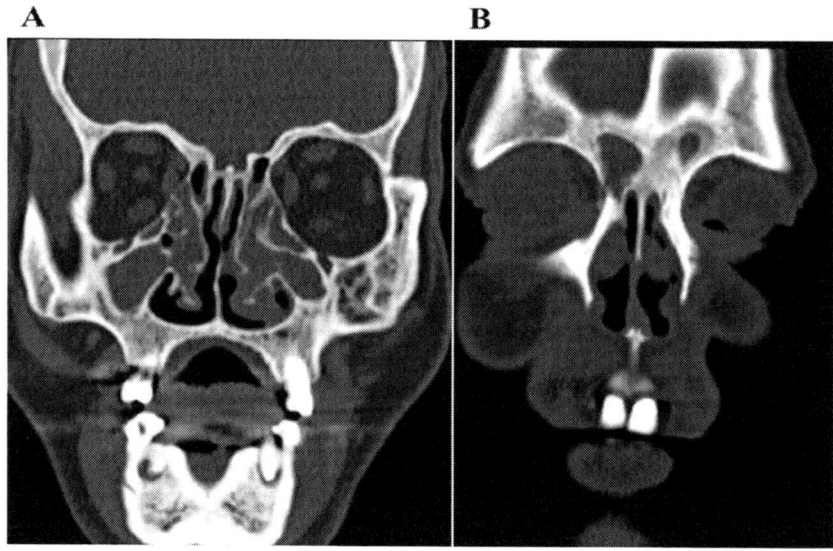

Figure 5. A) Sinus Hypoplasia and B) Pansinusitis in PCD.

As mentioned in the children section, the bacteriology of nasal secretions shows that the most frequent bacteria are *Haemophilus influenzae,* followed by *Streptococcus pneumoniae* and *Pseudomonas aeruginosa. Moraxella catarrhalis* and *Staphylococcus aureus* can also be present. However, when the sample is taken directly on the surgical bed by endoscopy, the most frequent is *Pseudomonas aeruginosa,* followed by *Haemophilus influenzae* and *Staphylococcus aureus* [48]. Longitudinal bacteriological studies show that the predominant flora is similar in children and adults, although in a different proportion, with *Pseudomonas aeruginosa* being more prevalent in adults, increasing this prevalence with age [36]. In addition, *Pseudomonas aeruginosa* develops a mechanism of adaptive mutations that facilitates chronic infection, turning paranasal sinuses into a reservoir that involves infection of the lower airways by different mechanisms, such as microaspirations by posterior rhinorrhea. Thus, adequate treatment of sinus infection by endoscopic surgery (ESS) and antibiotics, not only improves chronic rhinosinusitis (CRS) but also that of the lower airways, by eliminating *Pseudomonas aeruginosa* lower pathway infection for several months [36].

3.2. Pulmonary Clinical Manifestations

Wet cough and bronchorrhea are permanent and from birth. Although bronchiectasis can appear in infancy, they are almost universal by adulthood. Cylindrical or saccular bronchiectasis involves middle and lower lobes and lingula (Figure 6). The extent and severity of bronchiectasis increase with age, while lung function worsens, an estimated rate of 0.49% per year, calculated with FEV1 [34, 49].

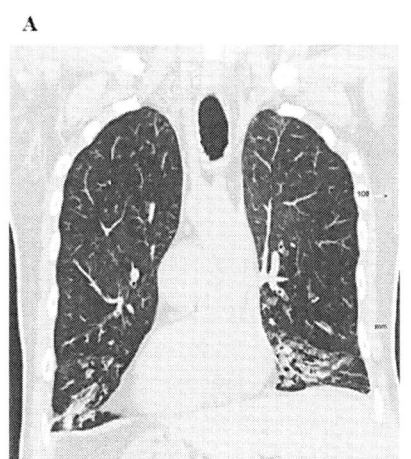
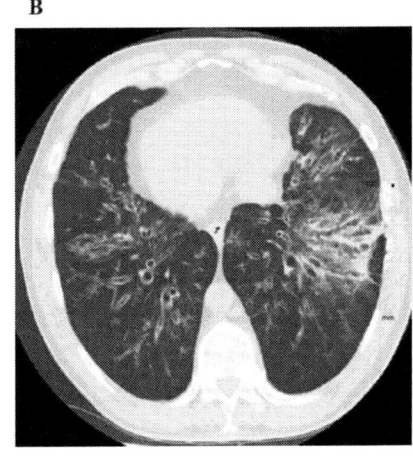

Figure 6. Bronchiectasis, atelectasis in middle and lower pulmonary lobes, and *situs inversus* in a patient with Kartagener's syndrome.

Other pulmonary tomographic findings in PCD are [50]: a) Mucous plugs are more commonly described in adults than in children, but in some children cohorts, they are present in 85% of the cases [51]. They are more frequently located in lower and peripheral lobes than in central ones [52]. b) The thickening of the bronchial wall is a universal finding of chest CT in children and adult PCD patients. Like in the rest of the findings, it is more frequent in middle and lower lobes and lingula [53]. c) Atelectasis related to PCD can be linear, lobar and segmental, being these last two more frequent (63%) in PCD than reported in CF and with a structural difference between them. Linear ones are less frequent (16%) in PCD and have not been reported in upper lobes [53]. d) Air trapping is described in almost all case series in the literature, one of the most recent PCD reports describes it in 33 of 39 CTs in expiration, which represents a prevalence of 85% [53].

Adult patients often have poor pulmonary function, ranging from mild to severe as a consequence of recurrent and chronic infection [54] Likewise, the older the diagnosis, the worse the lung prognosis. Older age at diagnosis was associated with an impaired FEV1 baseline ($r = -0.30$, $p = 0.01$) and increased *Pseudomonas aeruginosa* colonization ($p = 0.002$) [49].

3.3. Fertility Problems

Fertility problems are apparent in some adults. While some men have alive but immotile sperms, impaired ciliary function in the Fallopian tubes delays ovum transport in women. However, some patients are fertile [55], and more studies are needed to determine the prevalence of infertility in PCD. There have been many reports of ectopic pregnancy in patients with PCD but it is not clear if it is more common than in the general population [56, 57]. A recent study places infertility in 75% of men and 61% of women, correlating this infertility with certain ultra-structural and genetic defects of PCD [58]. Other recent studies have demonstrated a correlation between affected genes and fertility phenotypes [58].

3.4. Other Clinical Manifestations

Defects in the organs' laterality, either complete (situs inversus totalis, 46% of patients with PCD) or incomplete (heterotaxy, 6% patients with PCD)) are also characteristic of this syndrome, as a consequence of functional deficit of nodal cilia (Figure 7). In some patients, they are associated with cardiac malformations, so when having a patient with cardiac malformations and respiratory infections, a possible PCD should be suspected [59]. Lateral disorders are as important in PCD that some authors consider any organ-laterality defect (situs inversus totalis, situs ambiguous, or heterotaxis) as a major criteria for its diagnosis [60].

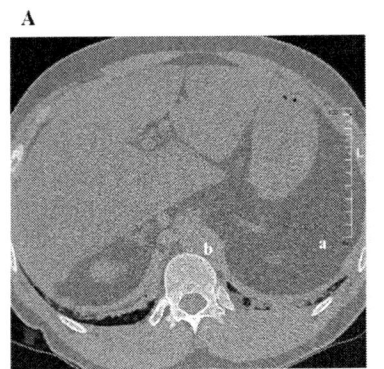 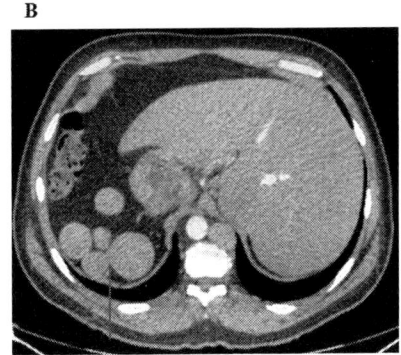

Figure 7. Two clinical forms of heterotaxy. A) Asplenia (a) and pancreatic hypoplasia (b). B) Polysplenia (arrow).

The association of PCD with other non-motile ciliopathies is rare, although two clinical conditions have been described in which PCD coincides with other alterations: Retinitis Pigmentosa (an inherited cause of blindness from retinal ciliary dysfunction) and Orofacial-digital Syndrome (including mental retardation, cranio-facial abnormalities, macrocephaly, digital anomalies, and cystic kidneys) are X-linked disorders involving ciliary genes, *RPGR* and *OFD1*, respectively [30, 61, 62].

Although common in murine models, neonatal hydrocephalus is rarely seen in PCD patients, and it is possibly related to ciliary dysmotility in brain ventricles [27].

3.5. Treatment

Currently, there is no treatment to restore ciliary motility and very few data from clinical trials about PCD management. Therefore, treatment is usually extrapolated from other diseases like cystic fibrosis and chronic rhinosinusitis. The aim of treatment is to delay the progression of lung disease while maintaining the patient's health, social, and psychological wellbeing [37].

The basic pillars of treatment are promoting mucociliary clearance, treating upper and lower respiratory tract infections with the most appropriate antibiotic (frequent sampling of respiratory secretion cultures), detecting and treating complications early, and optimizing treatment for otitis and rhinosinusal pathology [63].

It is recommended that these patients are followed up in a specialized clinic by a multidisciplinary team that includes pulmonologists, otolaryngologists, physiotherapists, nutritionists, and specialized nurses.

The recommended follow-up schedule based on the European guidelines and the United Kingdom National Health Service recommendations is summarized in Table 1 [64].

3.6. General Measures

Active and passive smoking, airway irritants, pollution, and cough suppressants should be avoided. Systematic vaccines should be administered in addition to influenza and pneumococcal vaccine.

A better nutritional status has been related to better lung function, so weight and height should be monitored, and nutritional support may be indicated in some cases [65].

Low vitamin D levels have been found to be common in PCD patients and may be related to an increased risk of chronic bacterial colonization and severity of bronchiectasis [66], so vitamin D levels should also be monitored.

3.7. Pulmonary Management

The main tools to enhance the clearance of secretions are respiratory physiotherapy and physical exercise.

Airway clearance should be performed daily (2 times a day), particularly during respiratory exacerbations. Its frequency can be reduced to once a week in those patients who are physically very active. Its main objectives are to reduce infections, atelectasis, bronchiectasis, and the progression of respiratory deterioration.

Airway clearance includes a series of techniques such as manual percussion, positioning, and positive or expiratory pressure devices. There are no studies to show whether one technique is better than others, so they should be individualized according to age, degree of involvement and personal preferences [67].

Physical exercise has been shown to be a better bronchodilator than beta-adrenergic agents in patients with PCD [66]. Regular exercise should be recommended to improve general wellbeing and perhaps assist in mucus clearance [37]. Nebulized treatments could increase mucus clearance, although evidence is poor in PCD [37].

Hypertonic saline increases airway's osmolarity and thus mucociliary clearance. This effect is widely proven in patients with cystic fibrosis. Only recently, a randomized study has been conducted in patients with PCD, failing to show a significant effect in comparison to isotonic saline. There was no significant improvement in quality of life scores, but there was some improvement in the perception scales of health [68].

Human recombinant DNase an enzyme that destroys the DNA of degraded neutrophils found in respiratory secretions, may improve their viscosity and clearance. However, unlike what happens in patients with cystic fibrosis, in randomized studies in adult patients with non-CF bronchiectasis, no benefit was seen in the quality of life, characteristics of sputum or lung function [69], and even in one study a worsening of FEV1 and an increase in pulmonary exacerbations was found [70]. For this reason, it is not usually recommended in PCD patients. It could only be considered on a case-by-case basis [37] as a small number of case reports have suggested a benefit [71].

There are no studies that support the routine use of other treatments such as bronchodilators, inhaled corticosteroids, or nebulized acetylcysteine. There is a prevalence of 8-10% of bronchial asthma associated with this disease, and in these cases, its use may be beneficial [72].

A randomized trial on the effects of azithromycin as an anti-inflammatory treatment (three days a week for 6 months) is currently awaiting publication of results [73].

Antibiotics should be used early and appropriately for respiratory infections' management according to the results of sputum culture or pharyngeal smears performed on patients. Monitoring the culture of sputum or cough swabs every 3-6 months is recommended [64]. Antibiotics are clearly indicated in the case of a respiratory exacerbation. There are no clear guidelines about treating or not bacterial colonization in asymptomatic patients; some authors suggest treating first isolates with at least 2 weeks of antibiotics in an attempt to eradicate them.

In adolescents and adults, it is common to isolate *P. aeruginosa*. Its treatment is similar to that established for patients with cystic fibrosis. A recent study [74] highlights the lack of consensus on this aspect in European centres, as 89% do not have a written guideline for *P.aeruginosa* eradication in patients with DCP. Eighty-seven percent of centres treat *P. aeruginosa* after the first isolation with an oral antibiotic (ciprofloxacin) together with (in 43% of cases) nebulized sodium colistimethate. For chronic infection, colistimethate (51% of cases) is the most used nebulized drug.

Sometimes surgical treatment may be indicated for bronchiectasis resection in case of severe localized bronchiectasis with recurrent febrile episodes or severe haemoptysis despite an aggressive medical treatment. In a retrospective study, 163 patients with lung resection were identified among a cohort of 2896 PCD patients [75]. Lung resection often was performed before PCD diagnosis and overall was more frequent in patients with delayed diagnosis. After lung resection, most lobectomised patients have poorer and continuing decline of lung function despite lung resection when compared to controls [75].

Patients with advanced disease may require oxygen therapy, non-invasive ventilation, or even a lung transplant [76].

3.8. ENT Treatment

Although we explain it extensively in adults, ENT problems start from childhood. More than 85% of patients report recurrent acute and serous otitis media, sometimes with decreased hearing, which usually improve progressively in adolescence and adulthood. For these cases, early treatment with antibiotics is recommended, and it is common to indicate ventilation tubes, since it may be associated with an increased risk of chronic otorrhea [5]. However, American guidelines advise tubes placement in cases of severe hearing loss since possible complications are treatable and the risk of presenting a secondary cholesteatoma (due to erosion of the ossicular chain) is reduced [77]. Another option in case of a marked decrease in hearing is the temporary use of hearing aids.

For treatment of chronic rhinosinusitis, daily nasal washes are recommended, and nasal anticholinergics and corticosteroids may be used, although there is usually no good response because, as in CF, inflammation is predominantly neutrophilic [78]. Sinusitis and polyposis treatment also involves an early use of antibiotics and, in recurring cases, surgical intervention may be assessed.

3.9. Specificities for Adult Management

As children management, treatments are based on evidence from other more common disorders. It is necessary to monitor airways disease, upper airways symptoms, and audiology. Consensus guidelines recommend treatment is based on combinations of antibiotics and airway clearance therapies [79]. And airway clearance should be improved by regular chest physiotherapy and physical exercise [80].

However, there are some aspects that we must take into account in adult patients. CT controls, both nasosinusal, and, above all, pulmonary, will no longer be restrictive, within the need to perform them only if necessary due to an aggravation of the disease or if the diagnosis has already been in adulthood. High-resolution computed tomography (HRCT) is a highly sensitive imaging modality for investigating PCD lung disease, and in particular, to detect bronchiectasis [81, 34, 52]. However, it involves larger radiation doses than the conventional X-ray procedure, and therefore its use in follow-up of chronic lung disorders is controversial [82]. Chest magnetic resonance imaging may be a valid alternative with a good-to-excellent agreement with HRCT findings [83, 84].

Bacterial flora changes in adults, making *Pseudomona aeruginosa* and other gram-negative organisms more prevalent. That is why it will be necessary to monitor patients through cultures of their bronchial and nasal secretions periodically. Culture results should guide antibiotic therapy during future respiratory exacerbations. When PCD patients are not responding to culture-directed antibiotics, physicians should consider additional nontuberculosis mycobacterial and fungal cultures, allergic bronchopulmonary aspergillosis testing (testing IgE levels evidence of aspergillus specificity) and bronchoscopy with bronchoalveolar lavage fluid cultures to guide antimicrobial therapy [30].

Surgical treatment of sinusitis in some patients may be indicated, especially if there have polyps that severely obstruct the nasal airway or if the infection is not controlled. In these cases, an improvement in the evolution of lower airway disease is observed [36, 85].

Although secretory otitis media and transmission hearing loss usually improve in adults, it is possible to need hearing aid or transtympanic drainage. Transtympanic drainage is controversial, but many times it is necessary, both to improve hearing and to decrease acute superinfections. Some studies highlight its obvious benefits, more effective than medical treatment, even in the child [86].

Genetic counseling and management should be offered to patients that want to have children, considering that it is an inherited disease. Intracytoplasmic spermatozoa injections could facilitate conception in males with immotile sperm [87]. In addition, in vitro fertilization and intra-uterine implantation could help female patients with PCD with decreased fertility [88].

3.10. Gene Therapy in PCD

Genetic correction of mutated PCD genes as a potential cure is gaining interest [37]. There are currently on-going research studies in cell culture and animal models about gene therapy [89], and also, several researchers are investigating targeted small molecule therapies [37].

In a study by Lai et al. [89] airway ciliated cells from two patients with PCD with DNAH11 nonsense mutations and altered ciliary beating frequency and pattern were collected. Repair of the genetic defect was performed ex vivo by site-specific recombination using transcription activator-like effector nucleases (TALENs). As a result, site-specific recombination and normalization of ciliary frequency and pattern occurred in 33% and 29% respectively.

In non-mobile ciliopathies, gene therapy experiments have been encouraging both in restoring ciliary function inner ear cells [90, 91] as in those of smell [92]. However, these therapies used fragments of adenovirus and lentivirus genome, without knowing what their effects would be on a living being over time.

Another important aspect to consider from the genetic point of view is that different mutations in the same PCD-associated gene may result in variable disease severity. Ciliary defects may be more common than previously appreciated, and subtle motile ciliary dysfunction could lead to persistent respiratory diseases or potentially modify other lung diseases in the general population [93].

Table 1. Clinical assessment for children with Primary Ciliary Dyskinesia. Modified from *Kuehni CE* et al., 2018. *"Management of primary ciliary dyskinesia: current practice and future perspectives"*. *ERS Monographs* 81:282–99

	At diagnosis	3-monthly	Annually	As needed
General care				
Height, weight	X	X	X	X
Vitamin D				X
Quality of life questionnaires			X	
Psychology assessment				X
Nutrition review				X
Lower airways				
Pulmonologist assessment	X	X	X	X
Physioterapist review	X	X	X	
Sample for culture	X	X	X	X
Chest radiograph	X		X	X
Spirometry	X	X	X	X
Chest CT (or consider MRI)				X
Bronchoscopy				X
Upper airways				
ENT assessment	X		X	X
Audiology	X		X	X
Other				
Echocardiogram	X			X
Abdominal ultrasound	X			
Fertility				X

4. DIAGNOSTICS

Because the symptoms described for PCD may also occur in other diseases, for example, allergies, immunodeficiencies or cystic fibrosis, it is recommendable to exclude these pathologies in patients with bronchiectasis of unknown cause or with repeated respiratory infections with chronic cough.

The diagnosis of primary ciliary dyskinesia is difficult, so referral of patients to a specialized centre is recommended. At present, diagnostic methods include [3]: nasal nitric oxide (nNO) levels (as screening test), study of ciliary beat frequency, and beat pattern with HSVM, ciliary ultrastructure by electron microscopy, cell cultures, immunofluorescence tests and genetic studies.

Determination of high levels of nNO can exclude PCD, although it may be inconclusive if clinical symptoms are very suggestive for this disease. Literature has reported cases of patients with a high flow rate of nasal nitric oxide [94]. For this reason, the European Guidelines suggest that when there is a high clinical suspicion of PCD, supported or not by the nNO levels, a functional study of the cilia (beat frequency and ciliary beat pattern) and ciliary ultrastructure study should be done; as well as immunofluorescence studies and genetics if available.

Early diagnosis may prevent progression of lung disease by delaying the onset of bronchiectasis and reducing the decline in lung function, as well as improving the management of rhinosinusitis and otitis symptoms [95]. In any case, the diagnosis of these patients is occasionally not determined until in adulthood.

Both the European Respiratory Society (ERS) and the American Thoracic Society (ATS) have recently developed diagnostic guidelines and recommendations for PCD (Figures 8 and 9). Due to the difficulty of performing the diagnostic tests and the high economic cost of them, the diagnosis of PCD is carried out in specialized centres.

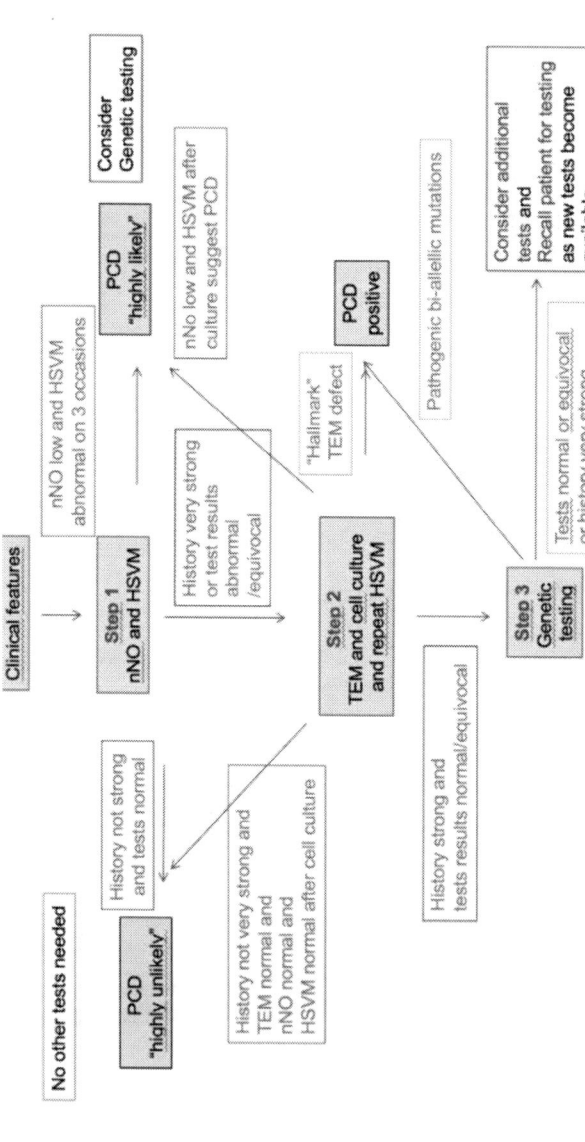

Figure 8. Adapted from ERS taskforce – PCD Diagnostic Guidelines – 2017 [3]. Nasal nitric oxide (nNO). High-speed video microscopy (HSVM). Transmission electron microscopy (TEM).

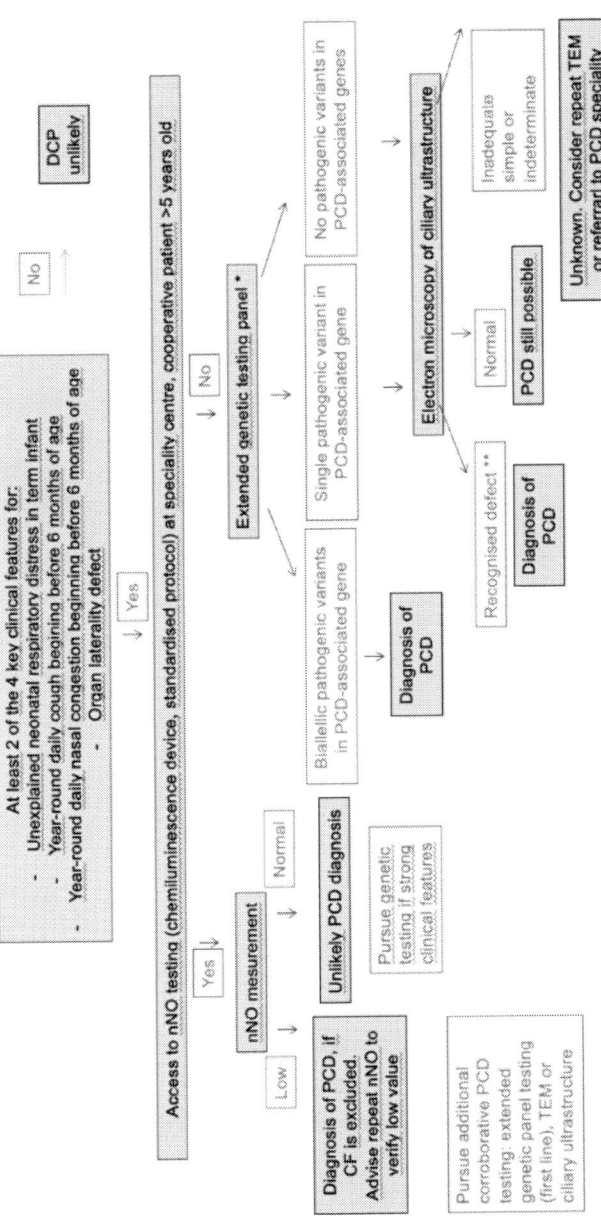

Figure 9. Adapted from ATS – PCD Diagnostic Guidelines – 2018 [96]. Nasal nitric oxide (nNO). Cystic Fibrosis (CF). Transmission electron microscopy (TEM). *: genetic panel testing for mutations in >12 disease-associated PCD genes, including deletion/duplication analysis. **: outer dynein arm (ODA) defect, ODA plus inner dynein arm (IDA) defects, IDA defect with microtubular disorganisation, absent central pair.

Confirming or discarding PCD diagnosis is not always clear and easy, and both guides propose a combination of tests to approximate accuracy. In fact, on multiple occasions diagnosis cannot be excluded or confirmed if clinical data are highly suggestive but tests are not. Therefore, the ERS guide classifies patients as "positive", "highly likely", or "highly unlikely."

There are important differences between the two guidelines. One of the most important is the role of nNO and genetics in the American Guidelines. Nasal nitric oxide is the first step (if it's available) for ATS Guidelines to continue or not the diagnostics tests, whereas it is only complementary for ERS Guidelines. In addition, values of nNO are considered low when <33 nL/min [3] by the European Guidelines and low when <77 nL/min [97] by the American Guidelines. Besides, genetic studies are considered the most important tests to diagnose PCD in the American algorithm, but not in the European ones, where it is only indicated in non-conclusive cases or positive cases if available.

Regarding cilia, functional studies, the study of ciliary motility wave (and cell cultures) is not considered a routine test for the American Guidelines and it is only performed in specialized centres in non-conclusive cases. On the contrary, it is the first step for the European ones. Conversely, electron microscopy analysis is considered in both guidelines. It should also be noted that, in none of the guidelines, immunofluorescence is yet not considered a diagnostic test within the diagnostic algorithm at present.

A recent study proposes some possible causes of these differences between the two guidelines. These are different healthcare and insurance systems (e.g., funding for HSVM *versus* genetic testing), different geography for access to tests, different government regulations for approval of new clinical diagnostic testing (e.g., medical device for nNO testing, certified labs for genetic testing) and different studies compiled to elaborate these guidelines. With regard to the considerable differences in both diagnosis pathways, this study claims working towards the development of an international diagnostic guideline for PCD [98].

4.1. Screening Tests

As previously mentioned, the diagnosis of PCD is complex and needs to be performed in specialized centers. In many cases, it's necessary to carry out a combination of tests for its diagnosis but still, they have their limitations and a conclusive diagnosis is not always obtained.

nNO measurement is used as a rapid non-invasive screening test for the diagnosis of PCD. Saccharin test and mucociliary clearance test with radioaerosol have used in the past, but the guidelines currently recommend the measurement of nNO [3] due to the disadvantages of the other two techniques.

Saccharin test consists in placing a 1-2 mm saccharin particle in the nose, approximately 1 cm behind the anterior end of the inferior turbinate, and then to control the time until the patient perceives sweet taste (normal time is one hour, approximately). Patient cannot sniff, cough, eat, or drink during the test. It requires collaboration and its result is very subjective, so it is rarely used in children [99]. It can't distinguish between primary and secondary ciliary dyskinesia, which is transient and due to an infection, allergy or inflammation of the airway.

Mucociliary clearance test with radioaerosol consists in the nebulization of albumin colloid labeled with 99-m technetium and subsequent measurements up to 120 minutes to calculate the mucociliary clearance. It is a very sensitive but not very specific test, so with this test, we can exclude the disease but not confirm it. Limitations of the test are the exposure of the patient to radiation and the need for collaboration, so it is not recommended to perform in children under 5 years or non-collaborating patients. Cough can invalidate the results, and the patient must return within 24 hours after the nebulization to continue the measurement [100].

Nitric nasal oxide and exhaled nitric oxide are decreased in PCD for reasons not yet clarified. Possible causes are 1) reduction of the biosynthesis of nitric oxide by decrease due to reduced activity of nitric oxide synthetase or 2) increase nitric oxide breakdown to its metabolites [101]. Nasal NO is more discriminative than exhaled NO, and it is a good screening test although difficult to perform in very young children under 5 years.

According to guidelines for diagnostic purposes, the technique must be performed with a stationary chemiluminescence analyzer and with the breathing maneuver of the velum closure technique [94]. A recent study has been published about nON measurement during tidal mouth breathing with rapid sampling spans (<2 seconds), which is feasible in children under 5 years of age or non-collaborating patients. This study suggests that the values obtained with this technique are also discriminative for the diagnosis of PCD [102]. There is not an established agreement on the values which are considered normal. European Guidelines considered low if the flow rate is <33 nL/min [3], and the American guidelines suggest a cut off of < 77 nL/min [97]. We have to consider that nNO can also be diminished in other diseases, although not so much as in PCD (cystic fibrosis, bronchiectasis of unknown cause, chronic sinusitis, Young's syndrome) [99]. Recent studies also put on alert that a low nNO measurement can be determined in case of respiratory infections and patients with adenoid hypertrophy, so the rate of the flow could be similar in this patients than in patients affected of PCD, so they recommend repeating the measurement in asymptomatic periods of time [103, 104]. The determination of high levels of nasal nitric oxide usually can exclude PCD, although it isn't a conclusive data if the clinical symptoms are very suggestive of the disease. Moreover, we can find in the literature reported PCD cases with elevated levels of nasal nitric oxide [94]. The sensitivity of the nNO for the diagnosis of PCD is 0.91 and the specificity is 0.96 [3].

4.2. High-Speed Video Microscopy

According to European Guidelines, the first test to be carried out on suspicion of PCD (with a low flow nNO rate or not) is the study of the ciliary beat frequency and pattern with HSVM. It is performed with a sample of ciliated respiratory epithelium that is obtained by brushing the nasal mucosa of the inferior nasal turbinate or septum with a small diameter bronchoscopy brush. This technique does not require anesthesia and only takes 2-3 seconds. An infection in the upper respiratory tract can cause damage to the respiratory epithelium (secondary ciliary dyskinesia). For this reason, it's recommended to postpone the test between 4-6 weeks after an acute respiratory tract infection.

The sample is placed in Medium 199 (pH 7,3), which contained antibiotic and antifungal solutions. Ciliated strips of epithelium are suspended in a chamber between a coverslip and a glass slide and they must be analyzed in the next 24 hours. Nevertheless, in one study it was found that ciliary beating accelerates during the first 3 hours after sampling with a plateau between 3 and 9 hours and then the speed falls in half from the initial starting at 12 hours, so they recommend performing the measurement within the first 9 hours [105]. The sample should be analyzed at a temperature of 37°C with an optical microscope with x100 interference lens and immersion oil mounted on an anti-vibration table. Ciliated strips have to measure more than 50 μm in length, devoid of mucus if it's possible.

Movement of cilia is recorded with a high-speed camera at 400-500 images per second and then can be played back the sequences at reduce frame rates or frame by frame. It is necessary to analyze the beat frequency and the pattern in different planes: lateral, towards the observer and vision from above [106, 107]. The reference range for the ciliary beat frequency is different according to the diverse studies (between 8.7 - 18.8 Hz [107, 108]), so it's recommended that each center has its own reference values. At least 10 ciliated epithelial edges with 10 cells in each of them should be evaluated in each sample, in addition to analyzing the pattern with at least 2 overhead visions (from above vision). Analysis of beat pattern is most important than ciliary beat frequency because 10% of patients with primary ciliary dyskinesia have a normal beat frequency but abnormal beat pattern [109].

There is a correlation between alterations in wave ciliary movements (frequency and pattern) and ultrastructure and specific genetics findings. For example, an abnormal hyperkinetic pattern has been correlated to a normal ultrastructure and it is caused by mutations in the *DNAH11* gene [110]. The ciliary beat frequency in cases of absence of external dynein arms is severely reduced or is static with minimal residual movement in most of the recordings. When external and internal dynein arms and regulatory complex factors are affected, cilia are static, and cases with mutations in *CCDC39* and *CCDC40* have an extremely stiff beat pattern. And when the defects are in the radial spoke head components, the beat frequency is normal or decreased but pattern (especially it can be observed in overheads edges) shows a circular motion in some areas. Mutations in *CCDC164* resulted in very subtle HSVM abnormalities with mild rigid pattern due to a decrease in amplitude [111].

With a normal result of HSVM, a normal ciliary beat frequency and pattern, in a patient with low clinical suspicion of PCD, no further complementary tests will be necessary. In case of low beat frequency, or dyskinetic beat pattern or a high clinical suspicion of primary ciliary dyskinesia, the sample must be analyzed with an electron microscope to see if there is any abnormality in the ciliary ultrastructure [112, 113]. A recent study by Rubbo et al. [114] showed that the HSVM study has a high sensitivity (1) and specificity (0.93) for the diagnosis of PCD.

In secondary ciliary dyskinesia, the abnormalities that we can find in the ciliary structure disappear when we repeat the tests (HSVM and ciliary ultrastructure) after performing a cell culture.

4.3. Transmission Electron Microscopy

TEM is actually one of the definitive PCD diagnostic tools given that it allows the unambiguous identification of ultrastructural defects causing the disease. TEM, when used properly, efficiently diagnoses more than the 70% of PCD cases. Thereby, some aspects regarding the technical procedures and the image analysis are crucial in order to diagnose efficiently the structural abnormalities involved in the cilia dysfunction characteristic of PCD.

Regarding specimens' collection, mucosa samples obtained from nasal curettage of the middle turbinate under topical anesthesia with lidocaine (2%) are preferred. These samples should ideally be fixed and processed for TEM, but if necessary, they can be suspended in bronchial epithelial culture medium supplemented with antibiotics and antifungals and sent to the pathology laboratory for analysis. Immersion in 2.5% glutaraldehyde in Sorensen buffer (pH 7.4, 0.03M) for 2h followed by incubation in 1% osmium tetroxide in the same buffer for 1h is the optimal fixing method to preserve ciliary ultrastructure. It also increases contrast enough to unequivocally determine the specific defect in the complex structure of the axonemal. Standard dehydration through graded acetone series enable specimens to be embedded in Epon 812 resin.

Evaluation and selection of the samples for morphometry analysis is another important point to be considered. This can be done by light microscopy study of semi thin sections stained with toluidine blue. Next, ultrathin sections stained with uranyl acetate and lead citrate can be examined under an electron microscope at 60 kV. Only cross-sections of ciliated areas are useful for ciliary ultrastructure examination. Sections form the tip of the cilium must be excluded. At least 100 cross-sectioned cilia must be examined per patient to avoid false positive diagnosis. The percentage of abnormalities must be calculated from the total number per cross-sections.

The most common structural abnormalities are peripheral microtubular alterations (extra, missing, or displaced microtubules), abnormalities of the central doublet, dynein arms, radial spokes, cilia orientation, and compound cilia. The absence of dynein arms (internal, external or both) can be considered when the mean of dynein arms is less than two per ciliary cross section [115]. Cilia orientation is normal if the variation of the ciliary axis is under 28 [116]. In our experience, the most common ultrastructure defects which can directly cause ciliary movement abnormalities are: ODA-defects (25-50%), combined ODA and IDA alterations (25-50%), IDA defects associated with microtubular disorganization (15%) and central microtubule pair defects (5-15%) [112, 117, 118]. The pathogenicity of isolated IDA alteration is controversial.

Regarding the incidence of axonemal alterations, the most frequent is the total lack of dynein arms. In some patients, the dynein arms persist, but the internal ones are uncommonly short. Abnormalities in peripheral microtubules, mostly some extra microtubules, are commonly observed in PCD patients. Other axonemal alterations are the presence of Compound cilia (quite common), central pair alterations, protrusions of the ciliary membrane and incomplete microtubular configurations that are present in a small number of patients [119].

It is important to highlight that the absence of outer dynein arms can be easily recognized, but the absence of inner arms is difficult to confirm because of their low contrast. The lack of the central pair [120] and absence of nexin [121] have been considered as possible congenital ciliary alterations, but it still needs to be confirmed. The total absence of dynein arms is associated with unmovable cilia, and the rest of the abnormalities in the ciliary structure give an inefficient mucociliary transport [112]. Regarding the displaced position of the central pair, it has a questionable pathological significance, and could also be due to technical aspects [122]–[126].

Another important limitation of TEM is that it not always allows to discriminate between primary or secondary dyskinesia. In general, alterations in the peripheral microtubules, as well as the compound cilia and the protrusion of the ciliary membrane, are common characteristics of secondary ciliary dyskinesia. A respiratory infection can cause transient dyskinesia associated with microtubular abnormalities that are reversible with appropriate treatment. The frequency of nonspecific or secondary acquired axonemal abnormalities has been reported to be significantly higher in patients with secondary ciliary dyskinesia than in patients with chronic respiratory infections and also only in 2–7% of healthy people [16, 116, 127]. However, we could not confirm this, nor other authors either [127, 115]. Alterations of ciliary ultrastructure, under the form of a deficit of dynein arms, must be considered diagnostic of the Kartagener syndrome in patients with chronic infections in the upper and lower airways and *situs inversus*. However, the ultrastructural normality does not imply the absence of PCD. These factors emphasize the need for a careful examination of a considerable number of cilia.

It is important to consider that the complexity of the technique and the exhaustiveness of the analysis can lead to false positive or negative diagnosis. This is important for ultrastructure defects affecting IDA that are, in most cases, difficult to identify. Central pair defects are characterized by a mix of both normal and abnormal cilia which involves the study of several cilia, sometimes more than 100 [118]. The above mentioned along with the complexity of the technique and the fact that some defects cannot be detected by classical TEM (particularly those affecting to the nexin link or central pair components, ciliary biogenesis or defects caused by mutations on *DNAH11*) could explain that the 20-30% of PCD patients have an apparently normal ultrastructure [118, 128].

4.4. Genetics

PCD is an inherited disorder characterized by a high allelic and locus heterogeneity. Thus, mutations in over 40 genes have been described as disease-causing (See Table 2). Its inheritance mode is mostly autosomal recessive, although X-linked forms have also been associated. PCD known genes screening allows the establishment of 65-70% families' genetic cause according to different published studies [37].

4.4.1. PCD Genes Classification

PCD genes are typically classified according to their protein location in motile cilia: outer dynein arm, inner dynein arm, microtubules' central pair, radial spoke, 96nm axonemal ruler, nexin-dynein regulatory complex, transport of these proteins, or different structures docking. PCD patients showing ultrastructural defects share the possibility of left-right laterality randomization during the embryogenesis. For this reason, approximately 50% of cases are associated with laterality defects, situs inversus, or heterotaxy. However, radial spoke, central pair and isolated nexin link defects coding genes, and reduction of multiple motile cilia generation gene mutations do not result in detectable ultrastructural defects on electron microscopy. Patients carrying mutations in these genes do not associate laterality defects and disease is presented as situs solitus.

Genes Coding for Outer Dynein Arm Components

Mutations in genes that encode outer dynein arm components result in outer dynein arms dysfunction. The most prevalent genes involved in PCD are included in this group. *DNAI1* was the first identified PCD gene, which accounts for approximately 9% of PCD patients. *DNAH5* is responsible for over 25% of PCD patients. Other genes included in this group are *DNAL1, DNAI2, NME8, DNAH11* and *DNAH9* which are responsible for less than 3% of cases.

Defects in *DNAI1, DNAI2, DNAL1, DNAH5* genes result in absence or deficiency outer dynein arms and immotile cilia. *DNAH9* defective cilia show absence of outer dynein arms, but only manifest subtle beating anomalies. Conversely, defects in the *NME8* gene result in variable ultrastructural phenotype, showing half of the ciliary cross-sections normal and the other half showing outer dynein arm defects. Mutations in *DNAH11* cause very rapid beat frequency with subtle abnormality in the ciliary waveform, reduced beating amplitude, and normal ciliary structure [37, 129].

Genes Coding for Proteins Involved in Outer Dynein Arm Docking and Targeting

Some PCD genes code for proteins involved in the outer dynein arm docking complexes, machinery that participate in the attachment of outer dynein arms to the outer doublets. These genes are *CCDC114, ARMC4, CCDC151,* and *TTC25*. When mutations in these genes are present, ciliary analysis by microscopy, transmission electron microscopy or immunofluorescence show absence of the outer dynein arms. Additionally, cilia are usually immobile [37]. The *CCDC103* gene also participates in the outer dynein arm targeting [130].

Genes Coding Cytoplasmic Proteins Involved in Assembly of Dynein Arms

Both outer and inner dynein arms are preassembled in the cytoplasm before being delivered to their final location in the microtubular doublets. Alterations in genes participating in the dynein arm protein assembly cause defects in the outer and inner dynein arms. In most of these cases, cilia are immotile and outer, or inner dynein arms are absent. These PCD genes are: *LRRC6, DNAAF1-6* (DyNein Axonemal Assembly Factors), *SPAG1, ZMYND10, CFAP298, CFAP300*. In some cases, some cilia motility can be observed (mutations in *DNAAF2* or hypomorphic variants in *DNAAF4*) [131, 132].

Genes Coding the 96nm Ruler Proteins

Along the ciliary length of the axoneme, a 96nm long unit repeat is observed in which four outer dynein arms and several inner dynein arms are anchored to the outer doublets. The proteins coded by *CCDC39* and *CCDC40* are essentials to this structure. Mutations in these genes show a reduction of amplitude and reduced bend, and deficiency of inner dynein arms proteins at the ultrastructure level [133, 134].

Genes Encoding Radial Spoke Proteins

Radial spoke components play an essential role in the regulation of activity of ciliary motility. Several genes encode for these proteins: *RSPH1, RSPH3, RSPHA4, RSPH9,* and *DNAJB13*. When mutations are observed in these genes, the absence of radial spoke proteins are observed by microscopy, while subtle ciliary beating abnormalities are present showing in most cases circular cilia motility [132].

Genes Encoding Central Pair Associated Proteins

Some proteins are associated with the central pair of single microtubules. To date, only mutations in two genes, *HYDIN* and *STK36*, have been described to cause central pair defects, resulting in very subtle abnormalities in the ciliary waveform and a normal ciliary ultrastructure with no microtubule disorganization, making difficult the diagnosis of these patients. In addition, *HYDIN*, the most prevalent gene in this subtype, presents a pseudogene (*HYDIN2*) due to an interchromosomal duplication, what difficult the genetic study due to its high homology [37].

Genes Coding Nexin-Dynein Regulator Complex Proteins

The nexin-dynein regulatory complexes connect the adjacent doublets to stabilize the peripheral ring. Genetic defects in genes encoding these proteins have been described in *DRC1, CCDC65,* and *GAS8* genes. In these PCD patients, ciliary beat patient is normal or subtle stiff, and the ciliary cross-section is usually normal [129].

Reduced Capacity to Generate Multiple Motile Cilia

Occasionally, PCD patients present a reduced generation of multiple motile cilia. In these cases, a lack of any motile cilia or residual cilia with normal motility is observed. Mutations in two genes, *MCIDAS* and *CCNO,* have been observed in these patients [135, 136].

Syndromes also Associating PCD

Two rare forms of X-linked syndromic PCD have been described. Mutations in *RPGR* cause an X-linked retinitis pigmentosa form that associates in some PCD patients' symptoms [61]. Genetic alterations in the *OFD1* gene have been detected classically in patients suffering from orofaciodigital syndrome. Over time, it has also been associated with other ciliopathies as X-linked intellectual disability, Joubert syndrome, Simpson-Golabi-Behmel syndrome type 2 and retinitis pigmentosa, being recently associated with PCD [62].

In recent years, in addition to the genes mentioned above, more genes have been related to PCD. Mutations in them have been identified in a small number of families, or functional studies should be performed to confirm their proposal as PCD genes. However, the evidences make them be proposed as candidate genes and are also listed in Table 2.

4.4.2. Genotype-Phenotype Correlation

Genotype-phenotype correlation in PCD patients is limited. However, in some cases, genetic and clinical relationships have been identified. Patients harbouring mutations in *CCDC39* and *CCDC40* manifest an earlier clinical presentation, worse lung function and lower body-mass indices that other PCD patients [23]. Defects in *RSPH1* associate with mild lung function impairment, low presentation of neonatal distress, and higher levels of nasal nitric oxide [137]. Patients presenting mutations in *CCNO* and *MCIDAS* manifest rapid deterioration in lung function with substantial bronchiectasis, hydrocephalus in 10% of cases and increased female infertility [28].

4.4.3. Genetic Analysis in PCD

In the last decade, new and improved technologies have emerged in the genetic diagnostic field. Of them, the Next Generation Sequencing (NGS) is the most widely used strategy for genetic diagnosis of diseases as PCD due to it enables a rapid, feasible and cost-effective method to perform genetic diagnosis of heterogeneous genetic and allelic diseases.

NGS can be employed by different forms. Targeted NGS panel including the known PCD genes is frequently the first used approach, providing a good coverage of screened genes, with a reduced or null incidental findings or variants of unknown significance. On the other hand, Whole Exome Sequencing (WES) is a high-throughput sequencing technique in which all coding regions of disease-related genes (termed clinical exome, mostly used in the diagnostic procedures) or all coding regions of all human known genes (whole human exome, mainly used in the research field) are sequenced. The WES sequencing, in either of these two ways, contributes to the swift identification of new PCD-causative genes and also to diagnose cases that could be mimicking the disease, allowing differential diagnosis in the same study.

Table 2. Genes associated with primary ciliary dyskinesia

Functional defect	Gene (Alias)	OMIM	Chromosome	Transcript Ref sequence	Protein Ref sequence	Number of exons	References
ODA	DNAH5	603335	chr5	NM_001369	NP_001360	79	[132]
	DNAH9	603330	chr17	NM_001372.3	NP_001363.2	69	[141]
	DNAH11	603339	chr7	NM_001277115	NP_001264044	82	[132]
	DNAI1	604366	chr9	NM_012144	NP_036276	20	[132]
	DNAI2	605483	chr17	NM_001172810	NP_001166281	14	[132]
	DNAL1	610062	chr14	NM_001201366	NP_001188295	8	[132]
	NME8 (TXNDC3)	607421	chr7	NM_016616	NP_057700	18	[132]
ODA docking/targeting	CCDC114	615038	chr19	NM_144577	NP_653178	14	[132]
	ARMC4	615408	chr10	NM_018076	NP_060546	20	[132]
	CCDC151	615956	chr19	NM_145045.4	NP_659482.3	13	[132]
	TTC25	617095	chr17	NM_031421.4	NP_659482.3	12	[132]
	CCDC103	614677	chr17	NM_213607	NP_004238	4	[130]
Preassembly Dinein Arms	LRRC6	614930	chr8	NM_012472	NP_036604	12	[132]
	DNAAF1 (LRRC50)	613190	chr16	NM_178452	NP_848547	12	[132]
	DNAAF2 (KTU)	612517	chr14	NM_018139	NP_060609	3	[132]
	DNAAF3 (c19orf51)	614566	chr19	NM_178837	NP_849159	12	[132]
	DNAAF4 (DYX1C1)	608706	chr15	NM_001033560	NP_001028732	10	[132]
	DNAAF5 (HEATR2)	614864	chr7	NM_017802	NP_060272	13	[131]
	DNAAF6 (PIH1D3)	300933	chrX	NM_001169154	NP_001162625	8	[132]
	SPAG1	603395	chr8	NM_172218	NP_757367	19	[132]
	ZMYND10	607070	chr3	NM_015896	NP_056980	12	[132]
	CFAP298 (C21orf59)	615494	chr21	NM_021254	NP_067077	7	[132]
	CFAP300 (c11orf70)	618058	chr11	NM_032930.2	NP_116319.2	7	[132]
96 nm Axonal Ruler Machinery	CCDC39	613798	chr3	NM_181426	NP_852091	20	[133]
	CCDC40	613798	chr17	NM_001243342	NP_060420	20	[134]
Radial Spoke	RSPH1	609314	chr21	NM_080860	NP_543136	9	[137]
	RSPH3	615876	chr6	NM_031924	NP_114130	8	[132]
	RSPH4A	612647	chr6	NM_001010892	NP_001010892	6	[132]
	RSPH9	612648	chr6	NM_152732	NP_689945	6	[132]

Functional defect	Gene (Alias)	OMIM	Chromosome	Transcript Ref sequence	Protein Ref sequence	Number of exons	References
	DNAJB13	610263	chr11	NM_153614.3	NP_705842.2	8	[132]
Central Pair	HYDIN	610812	chr16	NM_001270974	NP_001257903	86	[132]
	STK36	607652	chr2	NM_015690.4	NP_056505.2	27	[132]
N-DRC	DRC1 (CCDC164)	615288	chr2	NM_052952	NP_443184	17	[132]
	CCDC65	611088	chr12	NM_001286957	NP_001273886	8	[132]
	GAS8 (DIRC4)	605178	chr16	NM_001481	NP_001472	11	[132]
Reduced Cilia	MCIDAS	614086	chr5	NM_001190787	NP_001177716	7	[142]
	CCNO	607752	chr5	NM_021147	NP_066970	3	[135]
Syndromes associated with DCP							
RP	RPGR	312610	chrX	NM_001034853	NP_001030025	15	[61]
RP, JS, OFD, SGB Syndromes	OFD1	300170	chrX	NM_003611	NP_003602	23	[62]
Motilia Cilia defects And Laterality Defects. Candidate genes to DCP							
	DNAH8	603337	chr6	NM_001206927	NP_001193856	93	[143]
	DNAH1 (HDHC7)	603332	chr3	NM_015512.4	NP_056327.4	78	[144]
	LRRC56	618227	chr11	NM_015690.4	NP_056505.2	27	[145]
	MNS1	610766	chr15	NM_018365.2	NP_060835.1	10	[41]
	GAS2L2	611398	chr17	NM_139285.3	NP_644814.1	6	[146]
	AK7	617965	Chr14	NM_152327.5	NP_689540.2	18	[147]

ODA: Outer Dynein Arm; N-DRC: Nexin link Dinein Regulator Complex; Rp: Retinitis pigmentosa; JS: Joubert syndrome; OFD: Orofaciodigital syndrome; SGBS: Simpson-Golabi-Behmel syndrome.

Most of the pathologic alleles identified in PCD genes are point mutations, including missense, nonsense and small deletions o insertions, detected after the filtering of the DNA variants identified by NGS. However, a certain number of large rearrangements have also been detected in several genes as *DNAH5, DNAH11, DNAAF1, DNAAF4, CCDC40, DRC1 or ZMYND10* [138– 140]. For this reason, in order to perform an accurate diagnosis in PCD patients, the screening of large deletions or duplications should also be standardized after the search of point mutations. Software's based on NGS data have been developed to detect large rearrangements in sequenced genes (e.g., DECoN; www.icr.ac.uk/decon). They have the advantage that with the same technique (NGS), large rearrangements can be detected in addition to point mutations. Additional techniques are CGH-array or MLPA (Multiplex Ligation-dependent Probe Amplification), whose probe kits are available for the PCD genes *DNAH5* or *DNAI1* are commercially available.

PCD diagnosis is important for patients. The earlier recognition of disease allows the implementation of the appropriate treatment from the earliest age improving their quality of life. In 30-35% of PCD patients, the genetic cause of the disease is not identified after the genetic study of all known causative genes. It could be explained partially by the possibility that mutations could be located in non-screened regions of analyzed genes, such as deep intronic or regulatory regions. Or in a certain number of cases, the genes causative of the disease remains to be identified.

4.5. Immunofluorescence

Immunofluorescence (IF), consisting in the localisation of different cilia proteins in human respiratory cells by fluorescence or confocal microscopy (example shown in Figure 10), has been recently proposed as a technique to improve understanding of disease-causing genes and diagnosis rate in PCD [3, 96]. Nowadays, an important number of antibodies against different cilia proteins are available, including antibodies against proteins in ODA, IDA, radial spoke head and dynein regulatory complex proteins [3].

The methodology for IF staining of ciliated respiratory epithelial cells was described by Omran and Loges [148]. Human respiratory epithelial cells are sampled by nasal-brush biopsy and resuspended in cell culture medium (RPMI). The sample is then spread or dropped onto glass slides, air dried and stored at -80°C until use. Cells must be fixed using organic solvents or cross-linking reagents, such as paraformaldehyde (PFA) (i.e., incubation in 4%PFA for 15 min). Subsequently, permeabilisation of cells (i.e., incubation in 2% Triton X-100 for 15 min) is necessary to make antigens available for antibodies. Before the incubation of primary antibodies, it is necessary the blocking of unspecific antigens to avoid nonspecific binding (i.e., 5% skim milk at room temperature for 1 hour or 1% skim milk at +4°C overnight). Incubation with primary antibodies can be performed at room temperature for a few hours or overnight at +4°C. Incubation with polyclonal or monoclonal secondary antibodies labelled with fluorescent dyes is necessary for cellular sublocalisation of proteins [148].

Different studies presented IF as a technique to understand the downstream effect of mutations in different PCD-related genes [3, 60]. On this matter, Lucas et al. published, in the European Respiratory Society guidelines for the diagnosis of PCD, the literature results of the correlation between the PCD-causing genes and their associated findings by TEM and IF [3]. Therefore, IF has been used to study the defect in cilia proteins in cohorts of patients with a different range of genetic mutations, providing information of the pathogenicity of these variants. This was described in a study of PCD patients with radial spoke head defects [149]. It is important to take into consideration that IF analysis could detect abnormalities in cases with normal TEM defects but may provide a normal result if the analysed proteins still express in cilia axoneme, as described in cases with mutations in *DNAH11* [150].

IF has also been proposed as a new reliable diagnostic tool, although fewer results of IF accuracy have been published [3]. Several centres included in the international registry for PCD, which was launched in January 2014, are using IF to aid diagnosis in PCD [151]. In this registry, a defect in cilia proteins studied by IF was one of the diagnosis criteria for the recruitment of patients [151]. The first study using IF as a diagnostic tool, in a large cohort of patients suggestive of PCD and control subjects, identified DNAH5 mislocalisation in patients with an ODA defect previously described by TEM [152]. The same authors described the different cellular sublocalisation of DNAH5 and DNAH9 by IF, indicating the existence of two types of ODA [152].

A recent study by Shoemark et al. [153] presented the accuracy of IF in the diagnosis of PCD. The methodology applied in this study consists in a two-step incubation: one with acetylated α-tubulin antibody, to visualize cilia, and another with six labelled antibodies against proteins in cilia axoneme. Firstly, all samples were assessed with the primary antibodies: DNAH5 (an ODA component), DNALI1 (an IDA component) and RSPH4A (a radial spoke component). Secondly, only selected cases were assessed with a second round of antibodies: RSPH9 (a radial spoke component), RSPH1 (a radial spoke component) and GAS8 (a component of the nexin-dynein regulatory complex) (Figure 11). Using the described panel of antibodies, different results regarding the accuracy of IF as a diagnostic tool were published. First, IF correctly identified a mislocalisation or absence of target proteins in 35 patients with a confirmed ultrastructural defect by TEM. Second, IF diagnostic accuracy was studied in a cohort of 386 patients with symptoms suggestive of PCD. The technique successfully identified an absence of target proteins in 22 of 25 patients with PCD, whereas the remaining three patients were demonstrated to have mutations in genes (DNAH11 and HYDIN) with normal ultrastructure. Normal staining was observed in 252 cases in which PCD was considered highly unlikely. Third, IF provided a result in 39 of 71 cases with a previously inconclusive result in other diagnostic tests. Taking all these results into account, this study demonstrated that IF is a useful diagnostic technique and presents the same accuracy as well-performed TEM analysis, which is why the authors support IF as a routine diagnostic test for PCD, especially when TEM expertise or equipment is not available [153].

CASE 1. (CCDC40 mutant)

CASE 2. (RSPH4A mutant)

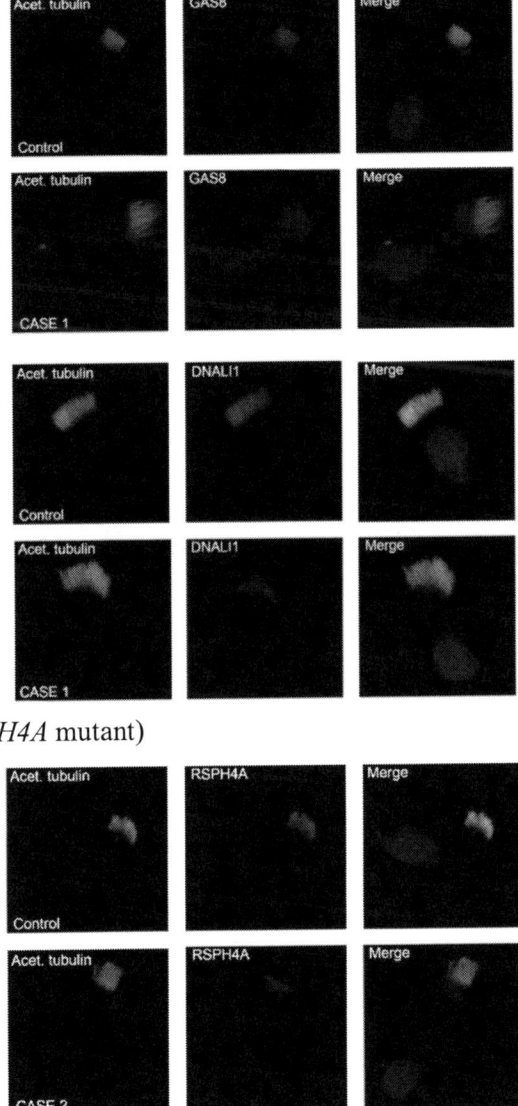

Figure 10. Example results of immunofluorescence technique in control subjects and patients with primary ciliary dyskinesia. *CASE 1:* patient with absence in GAS8 and DNALI1, explained by a homozygous pathogenic variant in *CCDC40*. *CASE 2:* patient with absence in RSPH4A. The first column shows cilia by acetylated α-tubulin (*green*); the second column shows the protein of interest (*red*); and the third column shows the final merged image with the nuclei stained with DAPI (*blue*).

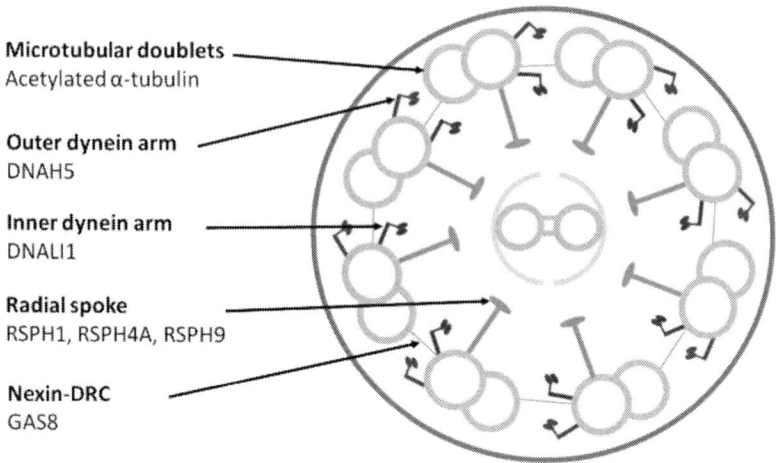

Figure 11. Cilia axoneme in transverse section indicating the ultrastructure parts and the target proteins by immunofluorescence. DRC = dynein regulatory complex.

The use of IF as a diagnostic test in PCD is believed to increase with more antibodies becoming available [3]. In the study by Shoemark et al. an improved first-antibodies panel with DNAH5, GAS8 and RSPH9 was proposed as a better approach to increase the diagnosis rate [153]. Therefore, it would be interesting to include, when commercially available, antibodies against proteins (DNAH11 [150], HYDIN [154], STK36 [155] and most recently SPEF2 [156]) with normal IF results using the previously described target proteins.

The main advantage of IF is the reduction of cost and time in comparison with TEM analysis, so IF may improve accessibility and accuracy of PCD diagnosis to a wider population of patients [153, 157]. Besides, IF also works on small samples [153], it is done in respiratory cells obtained by non-invasive brushings and dried samples in slides may be easily transported. Furthermore, secondary ciliary changes do not affect axonemal localisation of ODA components and this technique detects changes along the entire ciliary axoneme whereas TEM only studies a cross section of the cilia [148].

The major limitation of the IF analysis is that because of the use of primary antibodies directed to specific proteins, defects in unrelated proteins may be missed. Moreover, patients with partial defects or missense mutations have shown to have normal IF results [153]. As new genes and proteins related with PCD are discovered, the antibody panels may need to be revised and expand in the future for an accurate diagnosis [157].

In conclusion, IF seems to be a new reliable technique to study the molecular biology of cilia axoneme and improve the accuracy and diagnosis rate of PCD. However, validation studies are necessary to include this technique in the diagnostic guidelines [3, 96].

4.6. Cell Cultures

According to ERS guidelines, diagnostic of PCD mainly relies in the correct characterisation of cilia ultrastructure by TEM, cilia function by HSVM and genetics [3]. Secondary damage of ciliated nasal tissue is common in samples of PCD-candidate patients. This may be due to recurrent respiratory infections or to damaging tissue when taking biopsies. Secondary damage may give equivocal lectures of ultrastructure (TEM) and/or cilia function (HSVM) leading to false-positive results. Thus, it is necessary to distinguish between acquired from inherited abnormalities of cilia to give a proper diagnosis of PCD. Besides, scarce samples or samples of low quality (with numerous red cells and/or mucus) may lead again to mistaken results. TEM analysis needs a considerable amount of ciliated cells to be consistent and low amount of sampling may lead to false positives (21%) and false negatives [3]. Furthermore, HSVM analysis may not be reliable when there are very few ciliated cells. Also, temperature, pH changes and bacterial contamination may also affect the outcome of ciliated-cell samples [3] and therefore ciliary function may be analysed within a few hours after sample collection. Inconclusive or incomplete analyses may lead to demand repeated nasal brushings that would be uncomfortable for the patient and cause a delay in the diagnosis.

Ciliated-cell cultures may solve these pitfalls in PCD diagnosis. These cultures are directly derived from patients' nasal samples and show no secondary structural and functional abnormalities after ciliogenesis [158]. In particular, consensus guidelines on diagnostic of PCD by the European Respiratory Society strongly recommend repeating the HSVM (ciliary beat frequency, CBF) assessment after cell culture, particularly after air-liquid interfase culture (ALI), to improve diagnostic accuracy of HSVM [3].

As commonly known, airway nasal mucosa is a pseudostratified epithelium composed of ciliated cells, goblet cells and basal cells. Goblet cells secrete mucus, ciliated cells move this mucus thanks to their cilia, and basal cells (stem cells) differentiate to any type of epithelial cells to regenerate the airway nasal tissue. Basal cells are present in a small proportion in airway nasal respiratory tissue. The process of differentiation of basal cells to fully functioning ciliated cells leads towards formation of cilia (ciliogenesis), and is the basis of cell cultures applied to the study of PCD. Two different approaches to cell culture in PCD have been developed: suspension cultures and ALI cultures. Suspension cultures consist in 3D-cell cultures in monolayer or spheroids [117, 159], whereas ALI cultures consist in 2D-cell cultures exposed to air [160, 161].

Use of cell culture to improve diagnosis of PCD was first led by Jorissen et al. [117]. Briefly, they enzymatically dissociated biopsies of respiratory epithelium and cultured cells on collagen gel with supplemented growth medium for 3 weeks. Afterwards, a monolayer suspension cultures (3D-cultures), so-called spheroids, was produced. These spheroids rotated and/or migrated when they differentiated and ciliogenesis occurred. This first report consisted in the production of cell cultures originated from tissue biopsies and in assessment of CBF and ciliary coordination (continuous and active movement) in spheroids from more than 700 individuals [117]. After culture, ciliary immotility was present in 78% of PCD patients (66% before culture), but never in non-PCD patients (8% before culture); uncoordinated ciliary activity was present in all PCD patients (90% before culture) and in none of the non-PCD patients; and CBF was abnormal in 93% of PCD patients (80% before culture) and always normal in non-PCD patients. They concluded that, after culture, CBF analysis and, even more, coordinated ciliary activity (100% specific and sensitive) are highly reliable for PCD diagnosis [117].

Pifferi et al. [159] described a simplified method for cell cultures in suspension (spheroids). Basically, they centrifuged cell suspensions from nasal samples, resuspended pellet with culture medium and seeded the suspension in collagen-pre-coated culture wells. 24 hours later, samples were moved to another well to eliminate adherent cells and red cells. Cultures were incubated and maintained until ciliogenesis took place in aggregated floating cells forming spheroids. Ciliogenesis occurred after 21 days. With this simplified method, they investigated 9 doubtful cases (15%) of a series of 59 cases with pneumonia (ciliary motion analysis and TEM: 22% PCD, 63% non-PCD, 15% inconclusive) and concluded that 4 patients had PCD and 2 presented secondary defects, yet 3 remained inconclusive [159].

However, the 3D-culture approach usually does not provide enough ciliated cells to perform a new TEM analysis [159]. Based on alternative methods of ciliated-cell cultures, widely used in research, Hirst et al. [160] first developed and evaluated an ALI culture from nasal epithelia to study PCD in 187 samples. This method yielded far more cilia than the suspension technique and allowed evaluation of ciliary beat pattern (CBP), CBF and TEM analysis from both ciliated epithelia: the original brushing and the cultures. ALI culture methodology was adapted from Gray et al. [162] and has been developed and modified elsewhere [160, 161, 163, 164]. Briefly, this method consisted in 3 phases (Figure 12): basal-cell proliferation, basal-cell proliferation in inserts and airway culture. Cell suspensions were seeded on collagen-pre-coated culture plates for 2-7 days for basal cell proliferation. When confluent, basal cells were seeded on a collagen-coated transwell insert for 2 days, adding proliferation medium in both insert and plate. When confluent, proliferation medium was removed completely and ALI medium was carefully added basolaterally (exclusively on the plate) to create an airway culture and induce differentiation of basal cells. According to Hirst et al. [160], ciliogenesis should appear after 2-3 weeks, and optimal ciliary growth, considered of more than 10% of culture surface [160], after 4-6 weeks since exposure of cells to ALI. From here, cultures were removed with a spatula, washed, dissociated by gentle pipetting and finally recovered. A small portion may be used for HSVM (CBF and CBP), another portion for TEM [160], and the rest for other approaches (i.e., immunofluorescence), or even frozen for further *in vitro* analyses.

The results of Hirst et al. [160] show that more than half of the cultured biopsy-brushings (54%, 101/187) became ciliated and all allowed TEM and HSVM evaluations. Biopsies of 12 out of 28 patients already diagnosed with PCD could be cultured (43%) and showed similar CBP and TEM outcomes before and after culturing. The rest of samples (159) belonged to 90 patients suspected of PCD with low dyskinesia and to 69 with significant dyskinesia. ALI cultures were successful in 79% of patients with low dyskinesia and in 26% of patients with higher, and all confirmed secondary dyskinesia. These data indicate that the degree of damage is important for successful ALI cultures. In addition, cultures helped to exclude PCD in 8 patients with high dyskinesia in original biopsies. Besides, 6 out of 25 biopsies without cilia could be re-evaluated thanks to ALI cultures: all showed normal function and ultrastructure. In a second study, Hirst et al. [161], compared HSVM and TEM outcomes pre- and post-ALI cultures to assess robustness of this technique after observing changes in post-culture ciliary phenotype in some of their patients. They observed that in all PCD cases, dyskinesia remained unchanged or increased, whereas in non-PCD subjects, secondary dyskinesia decreased. They concluded that this exacerbation in cilia phenotype did not affect diagnosis of PCD and, in some cases, it may clarify it [161].

Ciliated-cell cultures are time consuming and need special equipment and experienced personnel [117, 159, 160]. In addition, different factors can limit both ALI and spheroid outcomes. Inherent respiratory infections and relatively few cells obtained (in brushing or after dividing the sample for different tests) increase the chance of failed cultures [117, 159]– [161]. Cultures started with a few cells have a low potential of differentiation and basal cells need more rounds to divide [160]. In practice, approximately only half of ALI cultures are successful (54%) and the rate of success is higher in biopsies with low dyskinesia [160]. This indicates that ciliogenesis in ALI cultures may also depend on degree of damage [160, 161]. On the contrary, spheroids have a higher percentage of success [159].

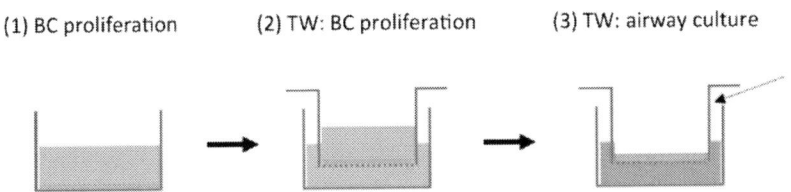

Figure 12. Air-liquid interface (ALI) cell culture steps. (1) basal-cell proliferation: cell suspensions are seeded on collagen-pre-coated culture plates for 2-7 days for basal cell proliferation. (2) When confluent, basal cells are seeded on a collagen-coated transwell insert for 2 days adding proliferation medium in both insert and plate. (3) When confluent, proliferation medium is removed and ALI medium is added basolaterally on the plate (see arrow) to create an airway culture and induce differentiation of basal cells. Ciliogenesis should occur after 2-3 weeks. BC: basal cells, TW: transwell insert.

However, advantages and possibilities of ciliated-cell cultures overcome their limitations. ALI cultures (a) produce enough cilia for a complete postculture analysis (TEM, HSVM, immunofluorescence, functional *in vitro* analyses, gene therapy, research), (b) are reliable as ciliary dyskinesia is maintained in PCD patients, (c) avoid re-biopsying in a certain amount inconclusive or incomplete samples and (d) can help in diagnosis of difficult cases. Human (and non-human) ALI cultures are widely used in diagnosis and research of respiratory diseases, including many investigations in respiratory tract biology, basic processes of respiratory diseases, gene therapy and drug administration [163, 165]. Spheroids have also been used in research and in attempts of gene therapy in PCD [166].

In conclusion, the use of cell culture from brush biopsy specimens may help to avoid re-sampling, reduce false-positive diagnosis in patients with secondary ciliary dysfunction, reevaluate difficult samples, confirm the diagnosis of less common phenotypes and evaluate new phenotypes of PCD.

CONCLUSION AND EXPERT COMMENTARIES

Cilia disorders are known as ciliopathies. Ciliopathies of primary cilia (non-motile ciliopathies) are responsible for diverse sensorial syndromes and deficits, such as smell (anosmia), hearing (sensorineural hearing loss), and vision (retinal degeneration) disorders. Primary ciliopathies are also responsible for conditions such as polycystic kidney, polydactyly, central nervous system malformations, developmental delay, heart, gonadal and craniofacial malformations as well as basal carcinomas. These features can occur in various combinations in a patient, leading to syndromes such as Usher (hearing and vision loss), Bardet Biedl, Alstrom, Joubert, Meckel Gruber, Senior Loken syndrome, and probably others that still unknown.

PCD is a motile ciliopathy caused by abnormal motile cilia. Primary ciliary dyskinesia is a congenital disease with an alteration in the ciliary motility biogenesis, also in its structure and function. Clinically, it manifests itself permanently and from birth as chronic sinopulmonary and otic infections, fertility problems (especially in men), and organ laterality disorders. It is an inherited, autosomal recessive disease, although there are forms linked to the X chromosome (two of them are syndromic). These syndromic forms can be considered as an association of motile and immotile ciliopathies and represent a very small proportion of PCD cases.

Organ's laterality alterations in PCD patients are consequence of cilia immotility of embryonic nodal cells, so the organs are distributed randomly. Organs laterality disorders have not direct consequences on health, but they do have indirect ones, given that thoracic-abdominal surgery in these patients requires precise preoperative studies and a great surgical experience. It is also important to highlight that, in PCD patients with laterality defects, cardiac malformations are more frequent, which means being attentive to our diagnostic study.

Patient's clinic is neonatal but nonspecific. That is why many patients are still diagnosed in adulthood. It is necessary to spread awareness of this disease so that health professionals, especially doctors, think about it and diagnose it early. Although not all studies conclude the same, most indicate that early diagnosis and treatment improve prognosis and quality of life of patients.

Presentation of unexplainable neonatal respiratory distress, especially if it is associated with any organ laterality alteration, with a family history of chronic respiratory problems and neonatal rhinitis, is highly suggestive of PCD and should be sufficient to initiate diagnostic studies.

As previously explained in this chapter, clinical symptomatology appears in new-borns and it remains present throughout the patient's life: productive cough and rhinorrhea are permanent. Secretory otitis media that will be able to also generate recurrent acute otitis media especially in childhood, will cause hearing loss in PCD patients. Exacerbations of otitis decrease over time, but hearing loss, which can be a mixture of transmission and sensorineural, persists in adulthood.

Similarly to other chronic diseases, PCD evolves with patients' growth. Lung lesions, especially bronchiectasis and atelectasis, appear and worsen with age. At the same time, lung function decreases, although the life expectancy of patients is affected to a lesser extent. The latest studies of genetic-clinical correlation explain the different evolution of lung function according to patients. In the upper respiratory tract, hypoplasia of paranasal sinuses in adults and pansinusal neutrophilic inflammatory involvement are very remarkable.

Over time, the quality of life of these patients is seriously affected, not only because of their health but also socially and because of the need for a chronic treatment. Bacteria that infect upper and lower respiratory tract are similar and vary as the disease is chronicled. Although *Haemophilus Influenzae* is the predominant microorganism, *Pseudomonas Aeruginosa* increases its presence over time and in many cases, chronically colonizes the respiratory tract. The infection of rhinosinusal pathways predisposes to that of the lower airways, although they generally follow a parallel course.

Adults have infertility problems, which affect a large part of men and fewer women. Literature review is inconclusive in terms of infertility rates. In most series, male infertility is 100%, while in women, there is only a decrease in fertility. However, in other series, not all men are infertile. Probably in the near future genetic variants that determine different cilia and flagella composition may explain these differences. Cases of women with PCD and ectopic pregnancies have been described, which are related to the deficient transport of the ovum through the cilia of the Fallopian tube, but the precise significance of this fact remains to be determined.

There is no definitive and unique diagnostic test. A typical clinical presentation, after discarding other diseases with conclusive diagnostic tests, such as cystic fibrosis or a congenital immunodeficiency, it is the starting point to initiate diagnostic studies. Depending on the health centre's availability, the diagnostic pathway begins by determining nasal nitric oxide, taking into account that false positives and negatives are possible.

The determination of mucociliary transport by saccharin cannot be considered useful because of its low specificity and the numerous artifacts that may interfere with its outcome. The study of mucociliary transport by radioisotope-labeled particles is more precise, but its specificity remains low, so it should not be considered a screening or diagnostic test.

Probably in the future, genetics will become the gold standard diagnostic test. However, since cilia composition involves more than 250 proteins, the number of genes involved is very large. Currently, genetic diagnosis is possible only in around 60% of patients. Therefore, it is necessary to have other diagnostic methods.

TEM gives a definitive diagnostic when findings are conclusive, especially if there are external and/or internal dynein arms defect. However, in 20-30% of the patients, they have a molecular alteration, not visible through TEM. Although it is becoming a very informative tool, to date, immunofluorescence is not considered a diagnostic test; it is only considered to support the determination of certain ciliary proteins defects.

The study of ciliary mobility using HSVM, as long as the ciliated epithelium sample meets the appropriate conditions and is evaluated by an expert, can be considered a very helpful diagnostic test in many cases. Ciliary beat pattern is the most informative aspect of ciliary mobility, as there are PCD cases with normal ciliary beat frequency. To analyse the ciliary pattern, it is very important to slow down recorded videos (up to 1/4 or 1/8). In cases of patients with a strong clinical history and a motionless or dyskinetic ciliary beat pattern, provisional diagnosis by HSVM may be considered sufficient to initiate treatment while completing genetic studies, TEM analysis or if these are inconclusive. However, we know that certain genetic mutations generate a ciliary dysmotility so subtle that it is difficult to distinguish from normal motility.

Thus, the PCD diagnostic pathway always starts with a compatible clinical history. In those centres that have it available, nNO measures is a first screening step. From our point of view, the first diagnostic test must be HSVM analysis, followed by TEM analysis and genetic testing. Many times, it is necessary to repeat sampling depending on the patient's state.

The complexity of diagnostics makes it necessary to refer a PCD suspicious to reference centres, with specialist in PCD professionals. These centres must be multidisciplinary since it is not only about diagnosis, but also the therapeutic management of patients. Difficulties caused by the lack of a standard gold test, necessity of specialists to carry out these tests, and funding availabilities for these services cause differences between countries.

Clinical management of patients requires lifetime medical care. Treatments should be adapted to clinical evolution, whereas respiratory physiotherapy is needed daily. Treatment with antibiotics is often needed and should be adapted according to the patient's clinical status and microbiological studies. Otitis media with effusion is common in patients with PCD, leading to recurrent acute otitis media, hearing loss, and potentially chronic suppurative otitis media even with cholesteatoma. Therefore, in some cases, surgical treatment (transtympanic drainage) is necessary. In children with hearing loss, hearing aids should be considered to prevent speech delay and educational compromise. Many adults, when surgical treatment of secretory otitis has not been sufficient, also need adaptation of hearing aids.

FUTURE PERSPECTIVES

One of the main goals is to achieve a better knowledge of clinical manifestations in order to prevent lung function deterioration, probably by studying differential inflammatory patterns in the respiratory tract. On the other hand, differentiated treatment diagrams according to the age and evolution of the disease in each patient must be developed (bronchopulmonary, rhinosinusal and otic).

Genetics will play a crucial role in the near future. It will be necessary to establish correlations between genetic mutations, ciliary mobility, ciliary ultrastructure and clinical manifestations of the disease. Knowing the genetic cause of the disease will allow an earlier and definitive diagnosis in all cases.

Gene therapy has already been tested with some success in olfactory and otic sensory ciliopathies. It has also been able to restore ciliary motility in a certain motile ciliopathy. In both cases, viral vectors have been used, which arouses suspicion because long-term effects are not known. They are experimental studies, but if it is possible at some time to be applied to patients, gene therapy will be able to restore ciliary motility, which means curring the disease.

REFERENCES

[1] Reula, A., et al., "New insights in primary ciliary dyskinesia," *Expert Opin. Orphan Drugs*, vol. 5, no. 7, pp. 537–548, Jul. 2017.

[2] Narang, I., R. Ersu, N. M. Wilson, and A. Bush, "Nitric oxide in chronic airway inflammation in children: diagnostic use and pathophysiological significance," *Thorax*, vol. 57, no. 7, pp. 586–589, Jul. 2002.

[3] Lucas J. S., et al., "European Respiratory Society guidelines for the diagnosis of primary ciliary dyskinesia," *Eur. Respir. J.*, vol. 49, no. 1, 2017.

[4] Baz-Redón, A., Noelia Rovira-Amigó, Sandra Camats-Tarruella, Núria Fernández-Cancio, Mónica Garrido-Pontnou, Marta Antolín, María Reula, Ana Armengot-Carceller, Miguel Carrascosa, Antonio Moreno-Gald, "Role of Immunofluorescence and Molecular Diagnosis in the Characterization of Primary Ciliary Dyskinesia," *Arch. Bronconeumol.*, vol. In press (, 2019.

[5] Barbato, A., et al., "Primary ciliary dyskinesia: A consensus statement on diagnostic and treatment approaches in children," *Eur. Respir. J.*, vol. 34, no. 6, pp. 1264–1276, 2009.

[6] Brown, J. M., and G. B. Witman, "Cilia and diseases," *Bioscience*, vol. 64, no. 12, pp. 1126–1137, 2014.

[7] Fliegauf, M., T. Benzing, and H. Omran, "When cilia go bad: Cilia defects and ciliopathies," *Nat. Rev. Mol. Cell Biol.*, vol. 8, no. 11, pp. 880–893, 2007.

[8] Popatia, R., K. Haver, and A. Casey, "Primary Ciliary Dyskinesia: An Update on New Diagnostic Modalities and Review of the Literature," *Pediatr. Allergy. Immunol. Pulmonol.*, vol. 27, no. 2, pp. 51–59, 2014.

[9] Siewart, A., "About a case of bronchiectasia in a patient with viscera situs inversus" *Berliner Klin. Wochenschrift*, vol. 41, pp. 139–141, 1904.

[10] Kartagener Manes, "On the pathogenesis of bronchiectasis," *Beitr. Klin. Tuberk. Spezif. Tuberkuloseforsch.*, vol. 31, no. 2, pp. 277–290, 1933.

[11] Afzelius, B.A, R. Eliasson, O. Johnsen, C. Lindholmer. "Lack of Dynein Arms in Inmotile Human Spermatozoa," *J. Cell Biol.*, vol. 66, pp. 225–232, 1975.

[12] Afzelius, B. A., "A human syndrome caused by immotile cilia," *Science*, vol. 193, no. 4250, pp. 317–319, Jul. 1976.

[13] Eliasson, R., B. Mossberg, P. Camner, and B. A. Afzelius, "The immotile-cilia syndrome. A congenital ciliary abnormality as an etiologic factor in chronic airway infections and male sterility," *N. Engl. J. Med.*, vol. 297, no. 1, pp. 1–6, Jul. 1977.

[14] Afzelius, B. A., P. Camner, R. Eliasson, and B. Mossberg, "On renaming the immotile-cilia syndrome," *Lancet (London, England)*, vol. 2, no. 8251. England, p. 870, Oct-1981.

[15] Afzelius, B. A., and B. Mossberg, "Immotile cilia," *Thorax*, vol. 35, no. 6, pp. 401–404, Jun. 1980.

[16] Rossman, C. M., and M. T. Newhouse, "Primary ciliary dyskinesia: evaluation and management," *Pediatr. Pulmonol.*, vol. 5, no. 1, pp. 36–50, 1988.

[17] Veerman, A. J., S. van der Baan, and W. Den Hollander, " [Disorders in mucociliary transport. Primary ciliary dyskinesia]," *Tijdschr. Kindergeneeskd.*, vol. 51, no. 6, pp. 185–192, Dec. 1983.

[18] Fischer, L., P. H. Burri, W. Bauer, R. Kraemer, and K. Sauter, " [How useful is the ultrastructural study of the cilia of the respiratory tract in

the diagnosis of an immotile cilia syndrome?]," *Schweiz. Med. Wochenschr.*, vol. 114, no. 18, pp. 610–619, May 1984.

[19] Mygind, N., M. Pedersen, and M. H. Nielsen, "Primary and secondary ciliary dyskinesia," *Acta Otolaryngol.*, vol. 95, no. 5–6, pp. 688–694, 1983.

[20] "*Orphanet.*" [Online]. Available: http://www.orpha.net/consor/cgi-bin/index.php.

[21] Rovira, S., "[Primary Ciliary Dyskinesia]" *Tratado Neumol. Infant.*, vol. 11, no. 1, pp. 991–1006, 2009.

[22] Kuehni, C. E., et al., "Factors influencing age at diagnosis of primary ciliary dyskinesia in European children," *Eur. Respir. J.*, vol. 36, no. 6, pp. 1248–1258, 2010.

[23] Davis, S. D., et al., "Clinical features of childhood primary ciliary dyskinesia by genotype and ultrastructural phenotype," *Am. J. Respir. Crit. Care Med.*, vol. 191, no. 3, pp. 316–324, 2015.

[24] Lucas, J. S., A. Burgess, H. M. Mitchison, E. Moya, M. Williamson, and C. Hogg, "Diagnosis and management of primary ciliary dyskinesia," *Arch. Dis. Child.*, vol. 99, no. 9, pp. 850–856, Sep. 2014.

[25] Kennedy, M. P., et al., "Congenital heart disease and other heterotaxic defects in a large cohort of patients with primary ciliary dyskinesia," *Circulation*, vol. 115, no. 22, pp. 2814–2821, 2007.

[26] Shapiro, A. J., et al., "Laterality defects other than situs inversus totalis in primary ciliary dyskinesia: Insights into situs ambiguus and heterotaxy," *Chest*, vol. 146, no. 5, pp. 1176–1186, 2014.

[27] Wessels, M. W., N. S. Den Hollander, and P. J. Willems, "Mild fetal cerebral ventriculomegaly as a prenatal sonographic marker for Kartagener syndrome," *Prenat. Diagn.*, vol. 23, no. 3, pp. 239–242, 2003.

[28] Amirav, I., et al., "Systematic Analysis of CCNO Variants in a Defined Population: Implications for Clinical Phenotype and Differential Diagnosis," *Hum. Mutat.*, vol. 37, no. 4, pp. 396–405, Apr. 2016.

[29] Mullowney, T., D. Manson, R. Kim, D. Stephens, V. Shah, and S. Dell, "Primary ciliary dyskinesia and neonatal respiratory distress," *Pediatrics*, vol. 134, no. 6, pp. 1160–1166, Dec. 2014.

[30] Shapiro, A. J., et al., "Diagnosis, monitoring, and treatment of primary ciliary dyskinesia: PCD foundation consensus recommendations based on state of the art review," *Pediatr. Pulmonol.*, vol. 51, no. 2, pp. 115–132, 2016.

[31] Zihlif, N., E. Paraskakis, C. Lex, L. A. Van De Pohl, and A. Bush, "Correlation between cough frequency and airway inflammation in children with primary ciliary dyskinesia," *Pediatr. Pulmonol.*, vol. 39, no. 6, pp. 551–557, 2005.

[32] Armengot Carceller, M., M. Mata Roig, X. Milara Paya, and J. Cortijo Gimeno, "[Primary ciliary dyskinesia. Ciliopathies]," *Acta Otorrinolaringol. Esp.*, vol. 61, no. 2, pp. 149–159, 2010.

[33] Sommer, J. U., et al., "ENT manifestations in patients with primary ciliary dyskinesia: prevalence and significance of otorhinolaryngologic co-morbidities," *Eur. Arch. Otorhinolaryngol.*, vol. 268, no. 3, pp. 383–388, Mar. 2011.

[34] Kennedy, M. P., et al., "High-resolution CT of patients with primary ciliary dyskinesia," *Am. J. Roentgenol.*, vol. 188, no. 5, pp. 1232–1238, 2007.

[35] Fitzgerald, D. A., and A. J. Shapiro, "Primary Ciliary Dyskinesia," *Paediatric respiratory reviews*, vol. 18. England, pp. 1–2, Mar-2016.

[36] Alanin, M. C., et al., "A longitudinal study of lung bacterial pathogens in patients with primary ciliary dyskinesia," *Clin. Microbiol. Infect.*, vol. 21, no. 12, p. 1093.e1-7, Dec. 2015.

[37] Lucas, J. S., S. D. Davis, H. Omran, and A. Shoemark, "Primary ciliary dyskinesia in the genomics age," *Lancet. Respir. Med.*, Oct. 2019.

[38] Goutaki, M., et al., "Clinical manifestations in primary ciliary dyskinesia: Systematic review and meta-analysis," *Eur. Respir. J.*, vol. 48, no. 4, pp. 1081–1095, 2016.

[39] Leigh, M. W., et al., "Clinical Features and Associated Likelihood of Primary Ciliary Dyskinesia in Children and Adolescents," *Ann. Am. Thorac. Soc.*, vol. 13, no. 8, pp. 1305–1313, 2016.

[40] Loges, N. T., et al., "Recessive DNAH9 Loss-of-Function Mutations Cause Laterality Defects and Subtle Respiratory Ciliary-Beating Defects," *Am. J. Hum. Genet.*, vol. 103, no. 6, pp. 995–1008, Dec. 2018.

[41] Ta-Shma, A., et al., "Homozygous loss-of-function mutations in MNS1 cause laterality defects and likely male infertility," *PLoS Genet.*, vol. 14, no. 8, p. e1007602, Aug. 2018.

[42] Sigg, M. A., et al., "Evolutionary Proteomics Uncovers Ancient Associations of Cilia with Signaling Pathways," *Dev. Cell*, vol. 43, no. 6, p. 744–762.e11, Dec. 2017.

[43] Behan, L., B. Rubbo, J. S. Lucas, and A. Dunn Galvin, "The patient's experience of primary ciliary dyskinesia: a systematic review," *Qual. Life Res.*, vol. 26, no. 9, pp. 2265–2285, Sep. 2017.

[44] Svobodova, T., J. Djakow, D. Zemkova, A. Cipra, P. Pohunek, and J. Lebl, "Impaired Growth during Childhood in Patients with Primary Ciliary Dyskinesia," *Int. J. Endocrinol.*, vol. 2013, p. 731423, 2013.

[45] C. E. Kuehni, M. Goutaki, M. Carroll, and J. S. Lucas, "Primary ciliary dyskinesia: the patients grow up," *The European respiratory journal*, vol. 48, no. 2. England, pp. 297–300, Aug-2016.

[46] Majithia, A., J. Fong, M. Hariri, and J. Harcourt, "Hearing outcomes in children with primary ciliary dyskinesia - A longitudinal study," *Int. J. Pediatr. Otorhinolaryngol.*, vol. 69, no. 8, pp. 1061–1064, 2005.

[47] Bequignon E., et al., "Critical Evaluation of Sinonasal Disease in 64 Adults with Primary Ciliary Dyskinesia," *J. Clin. Med.*, vol. 8, no. 5, May 2019.

[48] Moller, M. E., M. C. Alanin, C. Gronhoj, K. Aanaes, N. Hoiby, and C. von Buchwald, "Sinus bacteriology in patients with cystic fibrosis or primary ciliary dyskinesia: A systematic review," *Am. J. Rhinol. Allergy*, vol. 31, no. 5, pp. 293–298, Sep. 2017.

[49] Shah, A., et al., "A longitudinal study characterising a large adult primary ciliary dyskinesia population," *Eur. Respir. J.*, vol. 48, no. 2, pp. 441–450, 2016.

[50] Lizbet, C., and M. Pérez, "Chest imaging in the study of primary ciliary dyskinesia in children," *Neumol Pediatr*, vol. 14, no. 2, pp. 95–99, 2019.

[51] Jain, K., et al., "Primary ciliary dyskinesia in the paediatric population: range and severity of radiological findings in a cohort of patients receiving tertiary care," *Clin. Radiol.*, vol. 62, no. 10, pp. 986–993, Oct. 2007.

[52] Santamaria, F. et al., "Structural and functional lung disease in primary ciliary dyskinesia," *Chest*, vol. 134, no. 2, pp. 351–357, Aug. 2008.

[53] Tadd, K., et al., "CF derived scoring systems do not fully describe the range of structural changes seen on CT scans in PCD," *Pediatr. Pulmonol.*, vol. 54, no. 4, pp. 471–477, Apr. 2019.

[54] Marthin, J. K., N. Petersen, L. T. Skovgaard, and K. G. Nielsen, "Lung function in patients with primary ciliary dyskinesia: A cross-sectional and 3-decade longitudinal study," *Am. J. Respir. Crit. Care Med.*, vol. 181, no. 11, pp. 1262–1268, 2010.

[55] Frija-Masson, J., et al., "Clinical characteristics, functional respiratory decline and follow-up in adult patients with primary ciliary dyskinesia," *Thorax*, vol. 72, no. 2, pp. 154–160, 2017.

[56] Munro, N. C., et al., "Fertility in men with primary ciliary dyskinesia presenting with respiratory infection," *Thorax*, vol. 49, no. 7, pp. 684–687, 1994.

[57] Halbert, S. A., D. L. Patton, P. W. Zarutskie, and M. R. Soules, "Function and structure of cilia in the fallopian tube of an infertile woman with Kartagener's syndrome," *Hum. Reprod.*, vol. 12, no. 1, pp. 55–58, Jan. 1997.

[58] Vanaken, G. J., et al., "Infertility in an adult cohort with primary ciliary dyskinesia: phenotype-gene association," *The European respiratory journal*, vol. 50, no. 5. England, Nov-2017.

[59] Garrod, A. S., et al., "Airway ciliary dysfunction and sinopulmonary symptoms in patients with congenital heart disease," *Ann. Am. Thorac. Soc.*, vol. 11, no. 9, pp. 1426–1432, Nov. 2014.

[60] Damseh, N., N. Quercia, N. Rumman, S. D. Dell, and R. H. Kim, "Primary ciliary dyskinesia : mechanisms and management," *Appl. Clin. Genet.*, vol. 10, pp. 67–74, 2017.

[61] Moore, A., et al., "RPGR is mutated in patients with a complex X linked phenotype combining primary ciliary dyskinesia and retinitis pigmentosa," *J. Med. Genet.*, vol. 43, no. 4, pp. 326–333, 2006.

[62] Budny, B., et al., "A novel X-linked recessive mental retardation syndrome comprising macrocephaly and ciliary dysfunction is allelic to oral-facial-digital type I syndrome," *Hum. Genet.*, vol. 120, no. 2, pp. 171–178, 2006.

[63] Lobo, L. J., M. A. Zariwala, and P. G. Noone, "Primary ciliary dyskinesia," *QJM*, vol. 107, no. 9, pp. 691–699, Sep. 2014.

[64] Kuehni, L. J., CE., Goutaki M, Rubbo B, "Management of primary ciliary dyskinesia: current practice and future perspectives," in *ERS Monographs*, 2018, pp. 282–299.

[65] Goutaki, M., et al., "Growth and nutritional status, and their association with lung function: a study from the international Primary Ciliary Dyskinesia Cohort," *Eur. Respir. J.*, vol. 50, no. 6, Dec. 2017.

[66] Mirra, V., et al., "Hypovitaminosis D: a novel finding in primary ciliary dyskinesia," *Ital. J. Pediatr.*, vol. 41, p. 14, Feb. 2015.

[67] Schofield, L. M., A. Duff, and C. Brennan, "Airway Clearance Techniques for Primary Ciliary Dyskinesia; is the Cystic Fibrosis literature portable?," *Paediatr. Respir. Rev.*, vol. 25, pp. 73–77, Jan. 2018.

[68] Paff, T., J. M. A. Daniels, E. J. Weersink, R. Lutter, A. Vonk Noordegraaf, and E. G. Haarman, "A randomised controlled trial on the effect of inhaled hypertonic saline on quality of life in primary ciliary dyskinesia," *Eur. Respir. J.*, vol. 49, no. 2, Feb. 2017.

[69] Tarrant, B. J., et al., "Mucoactive agents for chronic, non-cystic fibrosis lung disease: A systematic review and meta-analysis," *Respirology*, vol. 22, no. 6, pp. 1084–1092, Aug. 2017.

[70] O'Donnell, A. E., A. F. Barker, J. S. Ilowite, and R. B. Fick, "Treatment of idiopathic bronchiectasis with aerosolized recombinant human DNase I. rhDNase Study Group," *Chest*, vol. 113, no. 5, pp. 1329–1334, May 1998.

[71] El-Abiad, N. M., S. Clifton, and S. Z. Nasr, "Long-term use of nebulized human recombinant DNase1 in two siblings with primary ciliary dyskinesia," *Respir. Med.*, vol. 101, no. 10, pp. 2224–2226, Oct. 2007.

[72] Fauroux, B., A. Tamalet, and A. Clement, "Management of primary ciliary dyskinesia: the lower airways," *Paediatr. Respir. Rev.*, vol. 10, no. 2, pp. 55–57, Jun. 2009.

[73] Kobbernagel H. E., et al., "Study protocol, rationale and recruitment in a European multi-centre randomized controlled trial to determine the efficacy and safety of azithromycin maintenance therapy for 6 months in primary ciliary dyskinesia," *BMC Pulm. Med.*, vol. 16, no. 1, pp. 1–11, 2016.

[74] Crowley, S., M. G. Holgersen, and K. G. Nielsen, "Variation in treatment strategies for the eradication of Pseudomonas aeruginosa in primary ciliary dyskinesia across European centers," *Chron. Respir. Dis.*, vol. 16, p. 1479972318787919, 2019.

[75] Kouis P., et al., "Prevalence and course of disease after lung resection in primary ciliary dyskinesia: a cohort & nested case-control study," *Respir. Res.*, vol. 20, no. 1, p. 212, Sep. 2019.

[76] Hayes, D. J., S. D. Reynolds, and D. Tumin, "Outcomes of lung transplantation for primary ciliary dyskinesia and Kartagener syndrome," *The Journal of heart and lung transplantation : the official publication of the International Society for Heart Transplantation*, vol. 35, no. 11. United States, pp. 1377–1378, Nov-2016.

[77] Campbell, R., "Managing upper respiratory tract complications of primary ciliary dyskinesia in children," *Curr. Opin. Allergy Clin. Immunol.*, vol. 12, no. 1, pp. 32–38, Feb. 2012.

[78] Ratjen F., et al., "Changes in airway inflammation during pulmonary exacerbations in patients with cystic fibrosis and primary ciliary dyskinesia," *Eur. Respir. J.*, vol. 47, no. 3, pp. 829–836, Mar. 2016.

[79] Abitbul R., et al., "Primary ciliary dyskinesia in Israel: Prevalence, clinical features, current diagnosis and management practices," *Respir. Med.*, vol. 119, pp. 41–47, 2016.

[80] Polineni, D., S. D. Davis, and S. D. Dell, "Treatment recommendations in Primary Ciliary Dyskinesia," *Paediatr. Respir. Rev.*, vol. 18, pp. 39–45, 2016.

[81] Eastham, K. M., A. J. Fall, L. Mitchell, and D. A. Spencer, "The need to redefine non-cystic fibrosis bronchiectasis in childhood," *Thorax*, vol. 59, no. 4, pp. 324–327, Apr. 2004.

[82] Brenner D. J., and E. J. Hall, "Computed tomography--an increasing source of radiation exposure," *N. Engl. J. Med.*, vol. 357, no. 22, pp. 2277–2284, Nov. 2007.

[83] Montella S., et al., "Assessment of chest high-field magnetic resonance imaging in children and young adults with noncystic fibrosis chronic lung disease: comparison to high-resolution computed tomography and correlation with pulmonary function," *Invest. Radiol.*, vol. 44, no. 9, pp. 532–538, Sep. 2009.

[84] Montella S., et al., "Magnetic resonance imaging is an accurate and reliable method to evaluate non-cystic fibrosis paediatric lung disease," *Respirology*, vol. 17, no. 1, pp. 87–91, Jan. 2012.

[85] Parsons D. S., and B. A. Greene, "A treatment for primary ciliary dyskinesia: efficacy of functional endoscopic sinus surgery," *Laryngoscope*, vol. 103, no. 11 Pt 1, pp. 1269–1272, Nov. 1993.

[86] Hadfield, P. J., J. M. Rowe-Jones, A. Bush, and I. S. Mackay, "Treatment of otitis media with effusion in children with primary ciliary dyskinesia," *Clin. Otolaryngol. Allied Sci.*, vol. 22, no. 4, pp. 302–306, Aug. 1997.

[87] Sha, Y.-W., L. Ding, and P. Li, "Management of primary ciliary dyskinesia/Kartagener's syndrome in infertile male patients and current progress in defining the underlying genetic mechanism," *Asian J. Androl.*, vol. 16, no. 1, p. 101, 2014.

[88] Lin, T. K., R. K. Lee, J. T. Su, W. Y. Liu, M. H. Lin, and Y. M. Hwu, "A successful pregnancy with in vitro fertilization and embryo transfer in an infertile woman with Kartagener's syndrome: a case report," *J. Assist. Reprod. Genet.*, vol. 15, no. 10, pp. 625–627, Nov. 1998.

[89] Lai M., et al., "Gene editing of DNAH11 restores normal cilia motility in primary ciliary dyskinesia," *J. Med. Genet.*, vol. 53, no. 4, pp. 242–249, 2016.

[90] Pan B., et al., "Gene therapy restores auditory and vestibular function in a mouse model of Usher syndrome type 1c," *Nat. Biotechnol.*, vol. 35, no. 3, pp. 264–272, Mar. 2017.

[91] McLean W. J., et al., "Clonal Expansion of Lgr5-Positive Cells from Mammalian Cochlea and High-Purity Generation of Sensory Hair Cells," *Cell Rep.*, vol. 18, no. 8, pp. 1917–1929, Feb. 2017.

[92] McIntyre J. C., et al., "Gene therapy rescues cilia defects and restores olfactory function in a mammalian ciliopathy model," *Nat. Med.*, vol. 18, no. 9, pp. 1423–1428, Sep. 2012.

[93] Horani A., and T. W. Ferkol, "Advances in the Genetics of Primary Ciliary Dyskinesia: Clinical Implications," *Chest*, vol. 154, no. 3, pp. 645–652, Sep. 2018.

[94] Simpson K., and M. Brodlie, "How to use nasal nitric oxide in a child with suspected primary ciliary dyskinesia," *Arch. Dis. Child. Educ. Pract. Ed.*, vol. 102, no. 6, pp. 314–318, 2017.

[95] Lucas J. S., et al., "Clinical care of children with primary ciliary dyskinesia," *Expert Rev. Respir. Med.*, vol. 11, no. 10, pp. 779–790, 2017.

[96] Shapiro A. J., et al., "Diagnosis of primary ciliary dyskinesia: An official American thoracic society clinical practice guideline," *Am. J. Respir. Crit. Care Med.*, vol. 197, no. 12, pp. e24–e39, 2018.

[97] Leigh, M. W., et al., "Standardizing nasal nitric oxide measurement as a test for primary ciliary dyskinesia," *Ann. Am. Thorac. Soc.*, vol. 10, no. 6, pp. 574–581, 2013.

[98] Shoemark, A., S. Dell, A. Shapiro, and J. S. Lucas, "ERS and ATS diagnostic guidelines for primary ciliary dyskinesia: similarities and

differences in approach to diagnosis," *Eur. Respir. J.*, vol. 54, no. 3, p. 1901066, 2019.
[99] Bush A., et al., "Primary ciliary dyskinesia: Current state of the art," *Arch. Dis. Child.*, vol. 92, no. 12, pp. 1136–1140, 2007.
[100] Marthin, J. K., J. Mortensen, and T. Pressler, "Pulmonary radioaerosol mucociliary clearance in diagnosis of primary ciliary dyskinesia," *Chest*, vol. 132, no. 3, pp. 966–976, 2007.
[101] Walker, W. T., A. Liew, A. Harris, J. Cole, and J. S. Lucas, "Upper and lower airway nitric oxide levels in primary ciliary dyskinesia, cystic fibrosis and asthma," *Respir. Med.*, vol. 107, no. 3, pp. 380–386, 2013.
[102] Holgersen, M. G., J. K. Marthin, and K. G. Nielsen, "Proof of Concept: Very Rapid Tidal Breathing Nasal Nitric Oxide Sampling Discriminates Primary Ciliary Dyskinesia from Healthy Subjects," *Lung*, vol. 197, no. 2, pp. 209–216, 2019.
[103] Marthin, J. K., M. C. Philipsen, S. Rosthoj, and K. G. Nielsen, "Infant nasal NO over time; natural evolution and impact of respiratory tract infection," *Eur. Respir. J.*, p. 1702503, 2018.
[104] Rybnikar, T., M. Senkerik, J. Chladek, J. Chladkova, D. Kalfert, and L. Skoloudik, "Adenoid hypertrophy affects screening for primary ciliary dyskinesia using nasal nitric oxide," *Int. J. Pediatr. Otorhinolaryngol.*, vol. 115, no. June 2018, pp. 6–9, 2018.
[105] Sommer, J. U., S. Gross, K. Hörmann, and B. a. Stuck, "Time-dependent changes in nasal ciliary beat frequency," *Eur. Arch. Oto-Rhino-Laryngology*, vol. 267, pp. 1383–1387, 2010.
[106] Jorissen M., and T. Willems, "Success rates of respiratory epithelial cell culture techniques with ciliogenesis for diagnosing primary ciliary dyskinesia," *Acta oto-rhino-laryngologica Belgica*, vol. 54. pp. 357–365, 2000.
[107] Chilvers, M. A., A. Rutman, and C. O'Callaghan, "Functional analysis of cilia and ciliated epithelial ultrastructure in healthy children and young adults," *Thorax*, vol. 58, no. December 2008, pp. 333–338, 2003.

[108] Ferkol T., et al., "Current issues in the basic mechanisms, pathophysiology, diagnosis and management of primary ciliary dyskinesia," *Eur. Respir. Monogr.*, pp. 291–313, 2006.

[109] Hogg, C. "Primary ciliary dyskinesia: when to suspect the diagnosis and how to confirm it," *Paediatr. Respir. Rev.*, vol. 10, pp. 44–50, 2009.

[110] Knowles M., et al., "Mutations of DNAH11 in patients with primary ciliary dyskinesia with normal ciliary ultrastructure," *Thorax*, vol. 67, pp. 433–441, 2012.

[111] Raidt J., et al., "Ciliary beat pattern and frequency in genetic variants of primary ciliary dyskinesia," *Eur. Respir. J. Off. J. Eur. Soc. Clin. Respir. Physiol.*, vol. 305404, no. 305404, p. in press, 2014.

[112] Chilvers, M. A., A. Rutman, and C. O'Callaghan, "Ciliary beat pattern is associated with specific ultrastructural defects in primary ciliary dyskinesia," *J. Allergy Clin. Immunol.*, vol. 112, pp. 518–524, 2003.

[113] Chilvers M. A., and C. O'Callaghan, "Analysis of ciliary beat pattern and beat frequency using digital high speed imaging: comparison with the photomultiplier and photodiode methods," *Thorax*, vol. 55, no. December 2008, pp. 314–317, 2000.

[114] Rubbo B., et al., "Accuracy of High-Speed Video Analysis to Diagnose Primary Ciliary Dyskinesia," *Chest*, vol. 155, no. 5, pp. 1008–1017, 2019.

[115] Lurie, M., G. Rennert, S. Goldenberg, J. Rivlin, E. Greenberg, and I. Katz, "Ciliary ultrastructure in primary ciliary dyskinesia and other chronic respiratory conditions: the relevance of microtubular abnormalities," *Ultrastruct. Pathol.*, vol. 16, no. 5, pp. 547–553, 1992.

[116] Nielsen, M. H., M. Pedersen, B. Christensen, and N. Mygind, "Blind quantitative electron microscopy of cilia from patients with primary ciliary dyskinesia and from normal subjects," *Eur. J. Respir. Dis. Suppl.*, vol. 127, pp. 19–30, 1983.

[117] Jorissen, M., T. Willems, and B. Van der Schueren, "Ciliary function analysis for the diagnosis of primary ciliary dyskinesia: advantages of

ciliogenesis in culture," *Acta Otolaryngol.*, vol. 120, no. 2, pp. 291–295, Mar. 2000.

[118] Papon J. F., et al., "A 20-year experience of electron microscopy in the diagnosis of primary ciliary dyskinesia," *Eur. Respir. J.*, vol. 35, no. 5, pp. 1057–1063, 2010.

[119] Carda, C., M. Armengot, A. Escribano, and A. Peydro, "Ultrastructural patterns of primary ciliar dyskinesia syndrome," *Ultrastruct. Pathol.*, vol. 29, no. 1, pp. 3–8, 2005.

[120] Stannard, W., A. Rutman, C. Wallis, and C. O'Callaghan, "Central microtubular agenesis causing primary ciliary dyskinesia," *Am. J. Respir. Crit. Care Med.*, vol. 169, no. 5, pp. 634–637, Mar. 2004.

[121] Carlen, B., S. Lindberg, and U. Stenram, "Absence of nexin links as a possible cause of primary ciliary dyskinesia," *Ultrastruct. Pathol.*, vol. 27, no. 2, pp. 123–126, 2003.

[122] Brauer, D. M. M., B. L. Viettro, D. M. M. Brauer, and B. L. Viettro, "[*Contributions of transmission electron microscopy to the diagnosis of ciliary dyskinesia*]" pp. 140–148, 2003.

[123] Sleigh, M. A., "Primary ciliary dyskinesia," *Lancet (London, England)*, vol. 2, no. 8244. England, p. 476, Aug-1981.

[124] Carson, J. L., A. M. Collier, and S. S. Hu, "Acquired ciliary defects in nasal epithelium of children with acute viral upper respiratory infections," *N. Engl. J. Med.*, vol. 312, no. 8, pp. 463–468, Feb. 1985.

[125] Afzelius, B. A., P. Camner, and B. Mossberg, "Acquired ciliary defects compared to those seen in the immotile-cilia syndrome," *Eur. J. Respir. Dis. Suppl.*, vol. 127, pp. 5–10, 1983.

[126] Pizzi, S., S. Cazzato, F. Bernardi, W. Mantovani, and G. Cenacchi, "Clinico-pathological evaluation of ciliary dyskinesia: diagnostic role of electron microscopy," *Ultrastruct. Pathol.*, vol. 27, no. 4, pp. 243–252, 2003.

[127] Buchdahl, R. M., J. Reiser, D. Ingram, A. Rutman, P. J. Cole, and J. O. Warner, "Ciliary abnormalities in respiratory disease," *Arch. Dis. Child.*, vol. 63, no. 3, pp. 238–243, Mar. 1988.

[128] Shoemark, A., M. Dixon, B. Corrin, and A. Dewar, "Twenty-year review of quantitative transmission electron microscopy for the

diagnosis of primary ciliary dyskinesia," *J. Clin. Pathol.*, vol. 65, no. 3, pp. 267–271, 2012.

[129] Kurkowiak, M., E. Zietkiewicz, and M. Witt, "Recent advances in primary ciliary dyskinesia genetics," *J. Med. Genet.*, vol. 52, no. 1, pp. 1–9, Jan. 2015.

[130] Panizzi J. R., et al., "CCDC103 mutations cause primary ciliary dyskinesia by disrupting assembly of ciliary dynein arms," *Nat. Genet.*, vol. 44, no. 6, pp. 714–719, May 2012.

[131] Horani A., et al., "Whole-exome capture and sequencing identifies HEATR2 mutation as a cause of primary ciliary dyskinesia," *Am. J. Hum. Genet.*, vol. 91, no. 4, pp. 685–693, 2012.

[132] Leigh, M. W., A. Horani, B. Kinghorn, M. G. O'Connor, M. A. Zariwala, and M. R. Knowles, "Primary Ciliary Dyskinesia (PCD): A genetic disorder of motile cilia," *Transl. Sci. rare Dis.*, vol. 4, no. 1–2, pp. 51–75, 2019.

[133] Merveille A. C., et al., "CCDC39 is required for assembly of inner dynein arms and the dynein regulatory complex and for normal ciliary motility in humans and dogs," *Nat. Genet.*, vol. 43, no. 1, pp. 72–78, 2011.

[134] Becker-Heck A., et al., "The coiled-coil domain containing protein CCDC40 is essentioal for morile cilia function and left-right axis formation," *Nat. Genet.*, vol. 43, no. 1, pp. 79–84, 2011.

[135] Wallmeier J., et al., "Mutations in CCNO result in congenital mucociliary clearance disorder with reduced generation of multiple motile cilia," *Nat. Genet.*, vol. 46, no. 6, pp. 646–651, 2014.

[136] Boon M., et al., "MCIDAS mutations result in a mucociliary clearance disorder with reduced generation of multiple motile cilia," *Nat. Commun.*, vol. 5, p. 4418, Jul. 2014.

[137] Knowles M. R., et al., "Mutations in RSPH1 cause primary ciliary dyskinesia with a unique clinical and ciliary phenotype," *Am. J. Respir. Crit. Care Med.*, vol. 189, no. 6, pp. 707–717, 2014.

[138] Loges N. T., et al., "Deletions and Point Mutations of LRRC50 Cause Primary Ciliary Dyskinesia Due to Dynein Arm Defects," *Am. J. Hum. Genet.*, vol. 85, no. 6, pp. 883–889, 2009.

[139] Raidt J., et al., "Ciliary beat pattern and frequency in genetic variants of primary ciliary dyskinesia," *Eur. Respir. J.*, vol. 44, no. 6, pp. 1579–1588, Dec. 2014.

[140] Morimoto K., et al., "Recurring large deletion in DRC1 (CCDC164) identified as causing primary ciliary dyskinesia in two Asian patients," *Mol. Genet. genomic Med.*, vol. 7, no. 8, p. e838, Aug. 2019.

[141] Fassad M. R., et al., "Mutations in Outer Dynein Arm Heavy Chain DNAH9 Cause Motile Cilia Defects and Situs Inversus," *Am. J. Hum. Genet.*, vol. 103, no. 6, pp. 984–994, Dec. 2018.

[142] Boon M., et al., "Primary ciliary dyskinesia: Critical evaluation of clinical symptoms and diagnosis in patients with normal and abnormal ultrastructure," *Orphanet J. Rare Dis.*, vol. 9, no. 1, pp. 1–10, 2014.

[143] Watson C. M., et al., "Robust Diagnostic Genetic Testing Using Solution Capture Enrichment and a Novel Variant-Filtering Interface," *Hum. Mutat.*, vol. 35, no. 4, pp. 434–441, 2014.

[144] Imtiaz, F., R. Allam, K. Ramzan, and M. Al-Sayed, "Variation in DNAH1 may contribute to primary ciliary dyskinesia," *BMC Med. Genet.*, vol. 16, no. 1, pp. 1–6, 2015.

[145] Bonnefoy S., et al., "Biallelic Mutations in LRRC56, Encoding a Protein Associated with Intraflagellar Transport, Cause Mucociliary Clearance and Laterality Defects," *Am. J. Hum. Genet.*, vol. 103, no. 5, pp. 727–739, Nov. 2018.

[146] Bustamante-Marin X. M., et al., "Lack of GAS2L2 Causes PCD by Impairing Cilia Orientation and Mucociliary Clearance," *Am. J. Hum. Genet.*, vol. 104, no. 2, pp. 229–245, Feb. 2019.

[147] Mata, M., J. Lluch-Estelles, M. Armengot, I. Sarrion, C. Carda, and J. Cortijo, "New adenylate kinase 7 (AK7) mutation in primary ciliary dyskinesia," *Am. J. Rhinol. Allergy*, vol. 26, no. 4, pp. 260–264, 2012.

[148] Omran H., and N. T. Loges, "Immunofluorescence Staining of Ciliated Respiratory Epithelial Cells," in *Methods in Cell Biology*, vol. 91, no. 08, Elsevier Masson SAS, 2009, pp. 123–133.

[149] Frommer A., et al., "Immunofluorescence Analysis and Diagnosis of Primary Ciliary Dyskinesia with Radial Spoke Defects," *Am. J. Respir. Cell Mol. Biol.*, vol. 53, no. 4, pp. 563–573, 2015.

[150] Dougherty G. W., et al., "DNAH11 Localization in the Proximal Region of Respiratory Cilia De fi nes Distinct Outer Dynein Arm Complexes," *Am. J. Respir. Cell Mol. Biol.*, vol. 55, pp. 213–224, 2016.

[151] Werner C., et al., "An international registry for primary ciliary dyskinesia," *Eur. Respir. J.*, vol. 47, no. 3, pp. 849–859, 2016.

[152] Fliegauf M., et al., "Mislocalization of DNAH5 and DNAH9 in Respiratory Cells from Patients with Primary Ciliary Dyskinesia," *Am. J. Respir. Crit. Care Med.*, vol. 171, pp. 1343–1349, 2005.

[153] Shoemark A., et al., "Accuracy of immunofluorescence in the diagnosis of primary ciliary dyskinesia," *Am. J. Respir. Crit. Care Med.*, vol. 196, no. 1, pp. 94–101, 2017.

[154] Olbrich H., et al., "Recessive HYDIN mutations cause primary ciliary dyskinesia without randomization of left-right body asymmetry," *Am. J. Hum. Genet.*, vol. 91, no. 4, pp. 672–684, 2012.

[155] Edelbusch C., et al., "Mutation of Serine/Threonine Protein Kinase 36 (STK36) Causes Primary Ciliary Dyskinesia with a Central Pair Defect," *Hum. Mutat.*, vol. 38, no. 8, pp. 964–969, 2017.

[156] Cindrić S., et al., "SPEF2 - and HYDIN -mutant Cilia Lack the Central Pair Associated Protein SPEF2 Aiding PCD Diagnostics," *Am. J. Respir. Cell Mol. Biol.*, vol. 23, pp. 1–59, 2019.

[157] Knowles M. R., and M. W. Leigh, "Primary Ciliary Dyskinesia Diagnosis Is Color Better Than Black and White ?," *Am. J. Respir. Crit. Care Med.*, vol. 196, no. 1, pp. 9–10, 2017.

[158] Jorissen M., and A. Bessems, "Normal ciliary beat frequency after ciliogenesis in nasal epithelial cells cultured sequentially as monolayer and in suspension," *Acta Otolaryngol.*, 1995.

[159] Pifferi M., et al., "Simplified cell culture method for the diagnosis of atypical primary ciliary dyskinesia," *Thorax*, 2009.

[160] Hirst, R. A., A. Rutman, G. Williams, and C. O'Callaghan, "Ciliated air-liquid cultures as an aid to diagnostic testing of primary ciliary dyskinesia," *Chest*, 2010.

[161] Hirst et al., "Culture of primary ciliary dyskinesia epithelial cells at air-li R. A., quid interface can alter ciliary phenotype but remains a robust and informative diagnostic aid," *PLoS One*, vol. 9, no. 2, 2014.

[162] Gray, T. E., K. Guzman, C. W. Davis, L. H. Abdullah, and P. Nettesheim, "Mucociliary Differentiation of Serially Passaged Normal Human Tracheobronchial Epithelial Cells," *Am. J. Respir. Cell Mol. Biol.*, 1996.

[163] Fulcher, M. L., and S. H. Randell, "Human Nasal and Tracheo-Bronchial Respiratory Epithelial Cell Culture BT - Epithelial Cell Culture Protocols: Second Edition," in *Epithelial cell culture protocols*, 2013.

[164] Lee, D. D. H., A. Petris, R. E. Hynds, and C. O'Callaghan, "*Ciliated Epithelial Cell Differentiation at Air-Liquid Interface Using Commercially Available Culture Media*," 2019.

[165] Stennert, E., O. Siefer, M. Zheng, M. Walger, and A. Mickenhagen, "In vitro culturing of porcine tracheal mucosa as an ideal model for investigating the influence of drugs on human respiratory mucosa," *Eur. Arch. Oto-Rhino-Laryngology*, 2008.

[166] Chhin B. et al., "Ciliary beating recovery in deficient human airway epithelial cells after lentivirus ex vivo gene therapy," *PLoS Genet.*, 2009.

In: Understanding Dyskinesia
Editor: Jan Dvořák
ISBN: 978-1-53618-502-7
© 2020 Nova Science Publishers, Inc.

Chapter 2

TARDIVE DYSKINESIA AND MENTAL ILLNESS: A SYSTEMATIC REVIEW

Alfonso Pedrós Roselló[1], Francesc Pascual Sanchis[1], Raquel Úbeda Cano[1], Begoña Pérez Longás[1], Dimitri Malventi Bellido[1] and Teresa Pedrós Diago[2]

[1]Psychiatry Department,
Lluís Alcanyís Hospital, Xátiva, Valencia, Spain
[2]Medicine Department,
CEU Cardenal Herrera University, Valencia, Spain

ABSTRACT

Tardive dyskinesia (TD) remains as an important clinical problem, causing severe limitations in daily life. It is a hyperkinetic movement disorder caused by the prolonged use of neuroleptics (NL), with a prevalence of 20-25%. It is classified as an extrapyramidal side effect induced by these drugs. Due to its severity, a proper assessment and monitoring of patients is necessary in order to avoid or reduce its intensity. However, with the emergence of new neuroleptics, new paths of hope have appeared, as the extrapyramidal profile of these molecules is more favorable than that of classical neuroleptics. The best way to minimize the risk of developing TD is to prevent it. This preventive approach should always be taken into account in patients with mental illness.

This chapter presents a systematic review of TD, covering the clinical manifestations, epidemiology, etiology, and an update on the therapeutic approach.

Keywords: tardive dyskinesia, mental illness, diagnosis, etiology, prevention, treatment

CLINICAL PRESENTATION

Tardive dyskinesia (TD) is an incapacitating movement disorder, associated to the prolonged use of neuroleptics (NL) or other drugs that can block the dopaminergic receptors (mainly D2), even though there have been case descriptions of spontaneous TD (Tenback and Harten, 2011). The term was first introduced in 1964 by Faurbye, emphasizing the delay between the beginning of treatment and the appearance of the abnormal movements.

On a clinical level, it is characterized by the insidious start of choreic, athetoid or rhythmical involuntary movements, that frequently affect the orofacial muscles and the upper extremities, although the muscles in the trunk and lower extremities can also be affected. Perioral movements are the most frequent, mainly lingual and masticatory, commonly accompanied by lip popping and tongue protrusion. Persistent blinking, cheek movement and smiling can also occur. The implication of the upper extremities involves finger movements, trembling, hand contraction and fist clenching. In more severe cases, the trunk is involved through rocking, torsion, and pelvic turns. Walk can be affected by the emergence of TD in the lower extremities (Frei et al., 2018). Furthermore, in advanced situations, the respiratory muscles can become affected, showing irregular breathing, aerophagy, and grunting. In some cases, DT can be accompanied by sensory phenomena such as paresthesia or pain (Waln and Jankovic, 2013).

In the fifth edition of the Diagnostic and Statistical Manual of Mental Disorders (DSM-5), TD is considered a motor disorder induced by medication, specifically the intake of NL for months (it might be a short period of time in the elderly). In some patients it can show after the suspension, change, or reduction of the dose of NL. This kind of dyskinesia is usually of limited duration, under 4-8 weeks. Dyskinesia with longer persistence is considered DT (A merican Psychiatric Association, 2013).

The intensity of TD is variable, it can be intermittent or persistent, patients can display almost imperceptible movements and, in other cases, very incapacitating ones. There can be fluctuations, alternating periods of spontaneous remission with periods of worsening. In addition, it tends to exacerbate with stress and to recede during sleep (Barberán et al., 2014).

Regarding the course of the disorder, if the NL is not suspended, the symptomatology shows an initial deterioration and after that a period of clinical stability. If the NL is suspended, symptoms can worsen initially and subsequently decrease. In the majority of patients with TD, the disorder persists for long periods of time and may even be permanent. Therefore, a complete remission of symptoms is uncommon (Cornett et al., 2017; Frei et al., 2018).

Differential diagnosis of TD has to be made with regard to the stereotyped movements that may appear in schizophrenia, spontaneous oral dyskinesia in advanced age, oral dyskinesia related to dental conditions, and oromandibular dystonia after a dental procedure or after the placement of a prosthesis (Frei et al., 2018).

EPIDEMIOLOGY AND RISK FACTORS

Incidence and prevalence of TD varies according to the consulted studies, probably due to methodological differences such as the study population or the definition of TD (D'Abreu et al., 2018).

The first reports on TD in psychiatric patients date back to the 1950's, shortly after NL were introduced. With prolonged use of typical NL, the risk of developing TD within 5 years was estimated to be 32%, 57% within 15 years, and 68% within 25 years (Glazer et al., 1993).

On the whole, the medium prevalence of TD after prolonged use of NL is 20% (Kane & Smith, 1982). The prevalence increases to 20-40% in patients who are hospitalized during long periods of time. Putting together the data from several studies published between 2004 and 2008, it is estimated that with prolonged use of NL the yearly incidence of TD is 7.7%, and 2-9% with atypical NL (Correll and Schenk, 2008). Therefore, the risk of developing TD with atypical NL is significantly lower than with typical NL (Cornett et al., 2017; Carbon et al., 2018).

Different studies show that the prevalence of TD is higher in patients treated with atypical NL who previously were using typical NL. The meta-analysis conducted by Carbon et al., (2017) showed that the prevalence of TD in patients who were treated with atypical NL with no previous exposure to typical NL was 7.2%, whereas in patients who had taken typical NL previously it reached up to 23.4%.

Recent studies, that included 11493 patients, identified a global prevalence of TD around 25.3% in patients who used neuroleptic medication (Fedorenko et al., 2015; Corell et al., 2018; Arunachalam et al., 2018; Vasan and Padhy, 2019).

Several risk factors for the development of TD have been found:

Age

It is the risk factor that gathers the most evidence. Advanced age is related to neurodegenerative progression and longer exposure to NL. With increasing age, the prevalence increases 1% yearly (Woerner et al., 1998). Thus, patients over 50 have 3 to 5 times more probability of developing TD than younger patients, and patients over 65 reach an increase of probability of 5 to 6 times (Kane et al., 1982). Age also influences the clinical presentation of TD, with bucco-lingual dyskinesia being the most frequent among older patients, and the dystonic presentations in younger patients (Venegas et al., 2003). Likewise, older patients show lower remission rates.

Gender

The evidence gathered is mixed. Initially, TD was considered to affect mainly women at a rate of 2:1 (Kane et al., 1988). Later studies suggested that both genders were equally susceptible to the development of TD. By contrast, current evidence shows that being female is a moderate risk factor, especially in postmenopausal women (Waln et al., 2013; Cornett et al., 2017). This might be explained by the fact that estrogens modulate the behaviors mediated by dopamine and have an anti-oxidative effect, and thus they may protect against the development of TD (Turrone et al., 2000). The severity of TD is higher in women, and the risk of TD in women as opposed to men increases in old age, suggesting a possible interaction between sex and age (Solmi et al., 2018).

African-American Race

Some studies suggest that African-american patients, especially older patients, show higher risk of TD compared to Caucasian patients (Tenback et al., 2009; Solmi et al., 2018). However, other studies have not found such differences (Ormerod et al., 2008).

Dosage and Duration of the Exposure to NL

The risk of TD increases in direct proportion to the daily dosage of NL, especially when it oscillates between 100-500mg per day of clorpromazin or an equivalent.

Previous Use of Typical NL

The previous exposure to typical NL might increase the risk of developing TD later with the use of atypical NL (Solmi et al., 2018).

Underlying Neurological Pathology

Some studies suggest the existence of a higher predisposition to develop TD in patients with neurological illness. Similarly, a higher predisposition to suffer TD has been found in patients diagnosed with AIDS. On the other hand, no higher prevalence has been found in patients with vascular dementia who require treatment with NL. Therefore, the available evidence is inconclusive (Venegas et al., 2003).

Negative Symptoms in Schizophrenia

Some studies find that, given a higher number of negative symptoms, there is a higher risk of TD (Telfer et al., 2011). Nevertheless, said association has not been consistently confirmed in other studies (Solmi et al., 2018).

Mood Disorders

Patients with comorbid affective disorders show higher probability of developing TD (Solmi et al., 2018).

Antecedents of Acute Extrapyramidal Symptoms Due to NL

The previous appearance of acute adverse movement reactions due to the use of NL, such as parkinsonism, acute dystonia or akathisia, among others, has been linked to a higher risk of later development of TD. (Kane et al., 1988; Tenback et al., 2006).

Abuse of Alcohol, Tobacco and Other Substances

The consumption of alcohol and other substances predisposes to develop TD (Potvin et al., 2009). Regarding tobacco, the existence of a positive correlation between the number of cigarettes consumed and the severity of TD is suggested (Diehl et al., 2009).

Diabetes Mellitus (DM)

The probability of developing TD and its severity is higher in patients with DM compared to patients without this pathology, combined with the fact that these patients can display dyskinesia, especially bucco-lingual, common to the diabetic illness (Ganzini et al., 1992).

Use of Anticholinergic Medication

Some anticholinergics, such as trihexifenidile, are broadly used in the case of acute dystonia. The prolonged use of these increases the relative risk of developing TD up to 6 times. Nevertheless, it is unknown if the use of the anticholinergic per se increases the risk of TD or if, actually, the acute dystonia does (Venegas et al., 2003).

"Drug Holidays"

Shorter duration and higher number of medication-free periods correlate with TD, increasing the risk of appearance up to 3 times (Branchey an Branchey, 1984).

ETHIOLOGY AND PHYSIOPATHOLOGICAL HYPOTHESIS

TD comes out as a result of prolonged exposure to drugs which act as antagonists to D2 dopaminergic receptors. It has been linked, first, to the use of typical NL, and, to a lesser extent, to atypical NL (Waln et al., 2013). Certain anti-emetics, such as metoclopramide, also cause TD (Rao and Camilleri, 2010). Similarly, there are some uncommon cases of TD linked to the use of other non-dopaminergic medications (Cornett et al., 2017), although there is insufficient consensus between different studies regarding the level of risk these drugs involve. This might be due to the existence of methodological differences and confusing variables, such as the intake of concomitant medications (D'Abreu et al., 2018).

With regard to TD's physiopathology, despite the fact that in the last decade multiple models and hypothesis have been suggested, it remains unclear. Current technology and multiple animal and human studies have increased our understanding of this side effect, but the definitive cause remains unknown. What is known is that the base of its physiopathology resides in a multifactorial mechanism which probably integrates the multiple models that have been studied so far. The oldest and most supported model is the neurochemical model, that tries to explain TD based on a receptor and neurotransmitter dysfunction; even though in the last decade there has been more interest in integrative theories, such as the genetic, the neural plasticity or the oxidative theory, which seem to explain this complex phenomenon in a more comprehensive way.

Neurochemical Models

Dopamine (DA) Availability and Hypersensitivity Theory

One of the most supported theories regarding the pathogenesis of TD is the chronic blocking of DA receptors. It is known that the abnormal movements require balance between the direct and indirect pathways to the basal ganglia, in connection to the cortex. Activating the direct pathway results in facilitating motor movements, since it stimulates the cortex on a net basis thanks to DA, through the D1 receptors. Instead, activating the indirect pathway has the final goal of reducing the speed and amplitude of the movements, expressing an inhibitory effect on the cortex through the D2 receptors. The chronic exposure to the NL creates a blockade of the D2 receptors, checking the inhibition of DA on the indirect pathway, generating cortical inhibition and as a result, hypokinesia. Furthermore, this chronic blockade of D2 receptors in the medial striatum increases the turnover of DA which, added to a compensatory rise in the synthesis of the D2 receptor (generally referred to as upregulation), leading to a state of hypersensitivity in the postsynaptic DA receptor (established by PET), causing a hyperkinesia (Silvestri et al., 2000; Turrone et al., 2003; Teo et al., 2012).

On the other hand, the receptors hypersensitivity to DA cannot explain why TD persists for years after abandoning the NL, since theoretically the DA receptors are not blocked and the DA should be able to link to its receptor.

DA-Gamma Aminobutyric Acid (GABA) Interaction Theory

This theory is supported by animal studies and states that there are GABA interneurons in the corpus striatum which regulate the balance of the direct and the indirect path to the basal ganglia (Gunne et al., 1984; Margolese et al., 2005; Gittis et al., 2011).

The GABA receptors have active spots for DA. Therefore, the GABA receptors situated in the striatum and the lateral globus pallidus are inhibited by the DA, while the ones located in the pars reticulata and medial globus pallidus are excited by DA. A lesion or dysfunction of this system could lead to a GABA hypo-function on the medial pallidus, which translates into hyperkinesia; and to a hyperactivity on the lateral pallidus, which induces parkinsonism. This would explain the coexistence of parkinsonism and hyperkinesia in TD.

Furthermore, genetic alterations of the glutamatergic system have been associated to this (Son et al., 2014), probably linked to previous observations of decrease of GABA levels in patients with TD (Thaker et al., 1987).

DA-Serotonin (5-HT) Antagonism Theory

In addition to DA and GABA, other receptors have been studied to determine the proneness of a drug to develop TD, as is the case of the 5-hydroxitriptamine receptors (5-HT2), especially the 5-HT2A and the 5-HT2C (Wolf MA et al., 1993).

These receptors are broadly distributed in the corpus striatum and it is thought that they are involved in the modulation of dopaminergic activity. Atypical NL show high blocking activity for the 5-HT2 receptor combined with a low occupation of the D2 receptor (or quick dissociation). These drugs might protect against TD due to the relative lack of stimulation of the D2 receptor (Glazer, 2000; Segman et al., 2001).

Quick Dissociation NL-Receptor Theory

Typical NL bind strongly and for a longer period of time to the D2 receptor, as opposed to the atypical NL, that display a much shorter blocking time. Atypical NL show a quick dissociation from the D2 receptor (12-24 hours after a single dose), which would explain the lower risk of TD (Seeman, 2010).

Noradrenergic (NA) Hyperactivity in TD

Recent studies have been bound to other, more promising directions, setting this neurotransmitter aside. There are several arguments in favor of the noradrenergic influence, even though they are based on older studies. One of them states the negative influence of treatments based on DA and NA recapture, such as amphetamines and methylphenidate, on TD; another underlines the action of NL not only on DA receptors but also NA receptors; and a third alludes to the effectiveness of drugs that inhibit NA activity, such as clonidine, in treating TD (Bacher and Lewis, 1980; Freedman et al., 1980).

Genetic Model

In clinical practice we see patients medicated with NL for years that do not develop TD while others, with the same treatment pattern, do. Furthermore, in this last group we find very different degrees of severity. These observations may be explained by individual genetic vulnerability or sensitivity. This increasingly fashionable theory is strengthening due to studies done in recent years which show a solid relationship between numerous genes and TD (Kulkarni and Naidu, 2003; Cho and Lee, 2012).

Several genes have been implicated in genetic predisposition, including those that code the D3 receptor, due to Ser9Gly polymorphism (Lerer et al., 2002); those that code the D2 receptor (Chen et al., 1997); the ones related to 5-HT2A serotonin receptors, being the T102C the gene associated to higher risk (Tan et al., 2001); the gene that codes manganese-superoxide-dismutase (Zhang et al., 2003); the one related to cathechol-O-methyltransferase (COMT) (Bakker et al., 2008); and several other genes with different degrees of association such as the GSK-3B (Souza et al., 2010). In addition, it has been described that disturbances in the P450 cytochrome (CYP2D6), responsible of changes in the drug's metabolism, may influence the risk of TD (Andreassen et al., 1997).

Currently there are research lines investigating the possible association of Neuroxin-1 (NRXN1) to TD (Lanning et al, 2017). NRXN1 is a transmembrane protein that interacts with Neuroligin (NLGN1) to create a calcium-dependent canal in the central nervous system (CNS), playing an important role in the GABA modulation in the synaptic cleft. This gene seems to be involved in the neuronal processes that develop or lead to TD. What we do know with certainty is that variations in the NRXN1 gene are related to multiple disorders, such as schizophrenia and autism, as well as alterations in white matter volume in the frontal lobe and intellectual disability (Bena et al., 2013; Todarello et al., 2014).

Oxidative Models and Structural Anomaly

Recently, the roles of oxidative stress or "neurodegenerative hypothesis" and the structural anomaly or "maladaptive synaptic plasticity" in the physiopathology of TD have achieved great momentum.

Maladaptive Synaptic Plasticity

According to this recent hypothesis, neural synapses have the capacity to increase or reduce their transmission based on learning, through different mechanisms, mediated by the increase of intracellular calcium. The chronic blockade of D2 receptors and their consequent hyper-sensitization, as stated in the first hypotheses in this chapter, cause a maladaptive neural plasticity in the cortical-striatal transmission, resulting in an unbalance between the direct and indirect paths of the basal ganglia. This theory is supported by the fact that this maladaptive neural plasticity may cause and perpetuate abnormal movements, even after interrupting the treatment with NL, as occurs in some of the patients with TD (Teo et al., 2012).

Neurodegenerative Hypothesis

This other model, which possibly combines with synaptic plasticity theory, is also supported by the irreversibility of symptoms after the interruption of treatment with NL. The defenders of this hypothesis suggest that the blocking of DA receptors lead to an increased availability of this neurotransmitter, which relates to an increase in the formation of free radicals due to monoamine-oxidase and auto-oxidation of the DA molecules, which transform into free radicals and quinines (Elkashe and Wyatt, 1999; Cho et al., 2012).

The increase in the production of free radicals, added to the deterioration of the anti-oxidative system, leads to an increase in oxidative stress, which in turn leads to neuronal damage and therefore the degeneration of the different neurotransmitter systems. This facilitates structural changes in the brain, including neuronal loss and gliosis in the basal ganglia. This neurolesion theory is based on the fact that these changes have been observed with chronic administration of NL in animal studies and in postmortem neuropathological exams of the brains of patients with TD (Kiriakakis et al., 1998).

Additionally, the oxidative stress hypothesis is supported by the finding that the activity of manganese superoxide dismutase (MnSOD), one of the main enzymes participating in the anti-oxidant defense mechanism, is heightened in TD patients' plasma, compared to subjects treated with NL without TD and healthy controls (Zhang et al., 2003). Other reinforcing aspects are that the enzymatic activity levels in patients with TD correlate directly with the severity of TD clinical symptoms and that the variations in the gene that codes the MnSOD are associated as well with TD (Hori et al., 2000).

In synthesis, there are multiple theories attempting to explain the origin of TD, although it is yet to be completely defined. The theories with the highest support and consensus found in recent studies are the genetic, the neuronal plasticity, and the neurodegenerative hypotheses; seen from a multifactorial and integrative point of view.

TARDIVE DISKINESIA TREATMENT APPROACH

Treatment of TD includes general measures for prevention, early detection, and treatment of potentially reversible cases. It also includes pharmacological treatment which, until 2017, was based on drugs lacking sufficient evidence. Nevertheless, with the arrival of the new inhibitors of the vesicular monoamine 2 transporter (VMAT2) (Correll and Carbon, 2017), a genuine revolution has occurred because they are the first drugs with a specific indication for TD.

General Measures

Before beginning treatment, the need for NL should be assessed and, if it is strictly necessary, administer the minimum effective dose for the minimum of time possible, constantly reevaluating the need to continue treatment. Patients should give informed consent to be treated with NL. Atypical NL such as quetiapine and clozapine are preferred against typical NL, but it should be noted that no NL is without risk and all of them can lead to TD (Lerner et al., 2013; Vijyakumar and Jankovic, 2016).

Additionally, prior to starting treatment, it is appropriate to explore presence of abnormal movements and register them in one of the existing scales, such as the AIMS (Abnormal Involuntary Movement Scale) (Guy, 1976), as well as to reassess patients treated with typical NL every 3-6 months, and every 6-12 months reassess patients with atypical NL (Niemann and Jankovic, 2018). The existence of abnormal movements should be reexamined every time a change is made in dosage or active principle.

Once treatment with NL is initiated, if TD emerges, the causing drug should be removed or reduced if possible. The reduction ought to be made gradually in order to avoid escalation of symptoms as well as of the underlying disorder (Mejia et al., 2010). The continued use of NL outside approved indications is discouraged. The addition of other drugs that might block DA receptors should be avoided although they have a different indication, as might happen with metoclopramide (Al-Saffar et al., 2019). No evidence has been found for the effectiveness of anticholinergics as preventive measures to avoid the appearance of TD (Jankovic and Clarence-Smith, 2011; Caroff et al, 2017).

Pharmacological Treatment

Dopaminergic Antagonists
We find two large groups of medications in this group.

DA Depletors

Their mode of action is to deplete DA inhibiting the VMAT in the presynaptic membrane of the nervous terminus, thus exposing the monoamines to monoamine-oxidase, resulting in depletion of the monoamine synaptic set (Jimenez-Shahed and Jankovic, 2013). There are two types of VMAT: VMAT1, which are found peripherally as well as in the CNS, their inhibition creates side effects such as bronchospasm, orthostatic hypotension, and gastrointestinal disorders; whereas VMAT2 are found only in the CNS, and their inhibition improves TD (Kenney and Jankovic, 2006; Lawal and Krantz, 2013). In the past, genetic typing was recommended prior to initiate this treatment, to avoid increase of side effects in slow metabolizers, however, different studies currently discourage this procedure (Mehanna et al., 2013).

Reserpine. It blocks VMAT1 as well as VMAT2, therefore causes a lot of side effects. It is not currently used with this indication.

Tetrabenazine (25-200mg/day distributed in 3 intakes). Selective inhibitor of VMAT1, same as valbenazine and deutetrabanzine, therefore much better tolerated than reserpine. It has been the most effective medication for the treatment of TD for many years, until new molecules appeared. In high doses it can cause depression, prolonged QT interval, lethargy, akathisia and parkinsonism.

Valbenazine (40-80mg/day in a single intake). The first drug approved by the Food and Drug Administration of the United States of America (FDA) with an indication for the treatment of TD. Several published studies show effectiveness, tolerability, and long-term security (O'Brien et al., 2015, Hauser et al., 2017).

Deutetrabenazine (12-48mg/day distributed in 2 intakes). The second drug approved by the FDA for the treatment of TD. It reduces the symptoms of TD compared to placebo in doses of 24-36mg/day and has much lower side effect rates than tetrabenazine (Anderson et al., 2017). Along with valbenazine, both are first treatment choice in monotherapy.

Neuroleptics

Increasing the dosage or introducing an atypical NL such as quetiapine, clozapine or aripiprazole in high doses have proved to be useful in the short term and for the control of emergent situations of involuntary movements. Nonetheless, their use is not recommended due to the recurrence of symptomatology in short periods of time and the high risk of producing akathisia and parkinsonism (Tamminga et al., 1994; Emsley et al., 2004; Peña et al., 2011).

Amantadine

It is a non-competitive blocker of the glutamate N-methyl-aspartate (NMDA) receptors. Two small studies informed of a statistically significant benefit in the improvement of the involuntary movements, even though the effect size was very small, it showed very few side effects (Angus et al., 1997; Pappa et al., 2010).

Anticholinergics

Medications like biperiden are usually not recommended for the treatment of TD. In addition, we have seen that the removal of these drugs leads to an improvement in the involuntary movements in patients taking it as a prophylaxis along with the NL (Caroff and Campbell, 2016; Citrome, 2017; Bergman and Soares-Weiser, 2018).

Cholinergic Agonists (Cholinomimetics)

None of the drugs in this group (rivastigmine, donezepil, galantamine, fisostigmine, choline) have shown any effectiveness in the treatment of TD in different studies (Tammenmaa et al., 2004).

GABA Agonists

Benzodiazepine. The efficacy of clonazepam is acceptable according to some papers, with doses from 80-240mg, however creates a tolerance that causes the beneficial affects to decrease rapidly. It is more effective for dystonic than dyskinetic symptoms (Thaker et al., 1990).

Non-benzodiazepine. The conducted research has not obtained evidence for valproic acid, baclofen or gamma-acetylene-GABA, and it may be possible that the side effects exceed the potential benefit of these drugs (Stewart et al., 1982; Alabed et al., 2011).

Gingko Biloba

After the administration of EGb-761 240mg/day, a standardized extract of this plant with strong anti-oxidant properties, patients displayed significant improvement compared to the placebo group, without finding any significant side effects (Zhang et al., 2011). However, another study did find hemorrhagic complications due to its strong antiplatelet effect (Pedroso et al., 2011).

Propranolol

It is a known B-blocker which in several isolated case studies and case series has demonstrated efficacy with doses from 30-160mg/day (Bacher and Lewis, 1980; Schrodt et al., 1982). Later it has been observed that its efficacy is related to the indirect increase it causes in the NL plasma levels (Silver et al., 1986).

Melatonin

A hormone produced by the pineal gland, it is known for its ability to eliminate free radicals and reduce oxidative damage in the CNS (Reiter and MAestroni, 1999). According to the studies carried out so far, the treatment of TD with melatonin at doses from 10-20mg/day is not clearly effective and new studies are needed to reach a conclusion due to the discrepancy of the obtained results (Shamir et al., 2001; Castro et al., 2011).

Others

Other multiple drugs have been studied for the treatment of TD, however none of them has shown any conclusive results. Among these we find: pyridoxine, vitamin E, omega3 fatty acids, zonisamide, levetiracetam, piracetam, nifedipine, buspirone, zolpidem, naltrexone, naloxone, insulin, estrogens, lithium, tryptophane.

Non-Pharmacological Treatment

Botulin Toxin

Small uncontrolled studies describe an improvement of the involuntary and stereotyped movements of the oro-bucco-lingual area after the injection of botulin toxin in the muscles that cause incapacitation (Jankovic, 2017). More relevant is its use in patients affected with tardive dystonia, especially blepharospasm and/or cervical dystonia (Tan and Jankovic, 2000).

Deep Brain Stimulation (DBS)

There is limited evidence on the efficacy of bilateral DBS of the nucleus pallidum (GPi-DBS) in the treatment of TD. But then again, according to a number of bibliographic revisions, it is an appropriate option when the TD is incapacitating and refractory to medical treatment (Spindler et al., 2013; Morigaki et al., 2016). It is a safe technique with little side effects and the outcome is maintained over 6 months (Meng et al., 2016).

Electroconvulsive Therapy

Some case series note improvement with this technique, however no firm conclusions can be drawn based on these studies (Manteghi et al., 2009; Yasui. Furukori et al., 2014).

TARDIVE DYSKINESIA, MENTAL ILLNESS AND QUALITY OF LIFE

Schizophrenia is a psychiatric disorder characterized by the presence of acute episodes followed by periods of stability. The majority of clinical guidelines recommend 1-2 year treatment after symptom remission of an acute episode. The risks of neuroleptic treatment include weight gain and metabolic and neurological disorders, among others. Given the magnitude of the adverse effects and the availability of strategies to deal with them, and the effectiveness of NL in relapse prevention, these medications have a positive risk-benefit balance during the first 1-2 years after the acute psychotic episode (Corell et al., 2018).

Nevertheless, the clinical guidelines do not provide systematic recommendations for the continuation or discontinuation of treatment beyond those years, despite warnings about the risks of relapse associated to their discontinuation. Current literature does not provide consistent evidence that proves the presence of irreversible functional or structural brain changes as a consequence of long term treatment with NL, other than TD (Corell et al., 2018). TD is a potentially irreversible and incapacitating syndrome (Samad et al., 2015; Arunachalam et al., 2018; Chen et al., 2018).

DSM-5 classifies TD as a motor disorder induced by medication, that might be developed after a short or long exposure to the use of medication, as well as after their suspension, change, or reduction. In all cases, TD should persist, at least, a month after suspending the medication to be able to establish the diagnosis (American Psychiatric Association, 2013).

The American Psychiatric Association (APA) recommends assessing the presence of motor disorders in patients before and after treatment with NL, which would allow to establish an early diagnosis and treatment, and thus increase quality of life for these patients (Diefenderfer et al., 2014; Arunachalam et al., 2018; Vasan and Padhy, 2019). APA advises to evaluate patients every 6 or 12 months, depending on whether they are being treated with typical or atypical NL. Those at high risk of developing TD, such as older patients or those who have suffered extrapyramidal side effects, should be examined every 3 or 6 months, according to whether they are taking typical or atypical NL (Diefenderfer et al., 2014; Yanan et al., 2017).

Generally speaking, prevention is the best method of battling TD. Before starting treatment with NL or other TD inducing drugs, clinicians should debate the risks with their patients and prescribe the lowest possible dose of a medication that potentially causes dyskinesia. Similarly, they should reevaluate the course of the illness and only maintain these medications for long periods of time if it is absolutely necessary (Vinuela and Kang, 2014; Barberán et al., 2014; Cornett et al., 2017).

Among patients with schizophrenia, the quality of life of those with TD is reduced in 12,3% (Yanan et al., 2017). The disability caused by the dyskinesia can be significant, in some cases leading to disfiguration, and cause isolation, shame, anxiety, depression and even stigmatization (Arunachalam et al., 2018).

On the other hand, TD has been linked to a higher degree of cognitive impairment in patients with schizophrenia, compared to those without dyskinesia (Wu et al., 2013; Arunachalam et al., 2018). Significant deficits have been found in the performance of a spatial working memory task, which is part of executive function (Pantellis et al., 2001).

TD entails a decline of social and occupational functioning, which increases the financial and social burden of mental illness (Diefenderfer, 2014; Caligiuri, 2015), which is also worsened by the lower therapeutic compliance of these patients (Yanan et al., 2017).

The motor disorders of patients with TD may affect one single area or multiple areas, in the latter case causing more severe abnormal movements and, consequently, a loss of mobility (Yanan et al., 2017). Among all areas affected by this condition, the orofacial is the main one (Yanan et al., 2017). The movements may precipitate oro-dental problems, including oral ulceration, speech difficulties, reduced salivation, and breaking of implants and prosthetic denture (Lumettiet et al., 2016; Arunachalam et al., 2018).

It has been suggested that patients with iatrogenic motor disorders, for instance parkinsonism or TD, compared to those who doesn´t suffer from them, have a higher dysregulation of the dopamine system. This may explain the relationship between the presence of abnormal hyperkinetic movements and the cognitive and negative symptoms of the psychotic illness, as well as its poor prognosis. In line with the above, motor disorders might act as predictors for psychosis in high risk patients (Van Harten et al., 2014; Martino and Morgante, 2017).

Moreover, a number of studies define the term of "tardive dysmentia." It is described as a behavioral syndrome similar to mania and it´s portrayed by affect, level of arousal, and social interaction disruptions. Studies link it to the severity of TD, the duration of the exposure to antipsychotics, and the physiopathology of schizophrenia (Lavania et al., 2013).

Furthermore, the subjective experience of patients with TD, obtained by a consulting group assembled by the Cochrane Group for Schizophrenia in

2016 is of special importance (Bergman et al., 2017). Individuals affected by dyskinesia are incapable of disguising its effects when they are in public. This, in turn, may have a very negative impact on their self-esteem and their ability to maintain social relationships. TD can be as impairing as psychosis itself.

A key topic is informed consent and the extent to which patients know about the adverse effects of NL. Lack of information prevents patients from being able to weigh pros and cons of taking the medication before starting the treatment. Informed consent is not only a key principle of treatment, but it also results in higher levels of adherence and satisfaction with it. Increasing the level of information given to patients does not lead to a direct decrease in the incidence of TD, but it does lead patients to feel more empowered and capable of accepting the consequences of any treatment.

None of the studies so far have explored the effectiveness of psychological therapies, peer support, and social interventions to help patients cope with symptoms. Coping mechanisms are highly important given the lack of effective treatments, particularly for those who experience these adverse effects chronically. The most debilitating aspects of living with TD come from social stigma and the negative impact it has on self-confidence.

Patients and their families consider that research regarding TD is, so far, limited. Firstly, they believed that patients needed more information about TD, in order to be able to make informed choices regarding medication. Secondly, they remark that there should be more emphasis on psychological and social interventions to deal with the symptoms of TD. Thirdly and lastly, it is stated that social stigma needs to be approached, since people's reactions to those who live with TD might be as inappropriate as the reactions to the symptoms of the mental illness.

In synthesis, a benefit-risk balance must always be kept in mind when administering NL, and a preventive approach should be taken regarding TD.

REFERENCES

Alabed, S., Latifeh, Y., Mohammad, H. A. and Rifai, A. (2011). Gamma-aminobutyric acid agonists for neuroleptic-induced tardive dyskinesia. *Cochrane Database Systematic Review*, 4, CD000203.

Al-Saffar, A., Lennernäs, H. and Hellström, P. M. (2019). Gastroparesis, metoclopramide, and tardive dyskinesia: Risk revisited. *Neurogastroenterology and Motility*, 00:e13617. https://doi.org/10.1111/nmo.13617.

American Psychiatric Association. (2013). *Diagnostic and statistical manual of mental disorders* (5th ed.). Washington, DC.

Anderson, K. E., Stamler, D., Davis, M. D., Gross, N., Hauser, R. A., Jarskog, L. F., Jimenez-Shahed, J., Kumar, R., Ochudlo, S. and Fernandez, H. H. (2017). Deutetrabenazine for treatment of involuntary movements in patients with tardive dyskinesia (AIM-TD): a double-blind, randomised, placebo-controlled, phase 3 trial. *Lancet Psychiatry*, 4, 595-604.

Andreassen, O. A., MacEwan, T., Gulbrandsen, A. K., Mc Creadie, R. G. and Steen, V. M. (1997). Non-functional CYP2D6 alleles and risk for neuroleptic-induced movement disorders in schizophrenic patients. *Psychopharmacology (Berl)*, 131, 174–179.

Angus, S., Sugars, J., Boltezar, R., Koskewich, S. and Schneider N. M. (1997). A controlled trial of amantadine hydrochloride and neuroleptics in the treatment of tardive dyskinesia. *Journal of Clinical Psychopharmacology*, 17, 88-91.

Arunachalam, M. A., Thavarajah, R., Nayak, D., Joshua, E., Krishnamohan, U. R. and Ranganathan, K. (2018). A Study on Drug-Induced Tardive Dyskinesia: Orofacial Musculature Involvement and Patient's Awareness. *Journal of Orofacial Sciences, 10,* 86–95.

Bacher, N. M. and Lewis, H. A. (1980). Low-dose propranolol in tardive dyskinesia. *American Journal of Psychiatry, 137*, 495-497.

Bakker, P. R., van Harten, P. N. and van Os, J. (2008). Antipsychotic-induced tardive dyskinesia and polymorphic variations in COMT,

DRD2, CYP1A2 and MnSOD genes: a meta-analysis of pharmacogenetic interactions. *Molecular Psychiatry, 13*, 544–556.

Barberán, M., Andreu, M., Sorribes, G. and Pedrós, A. (2014). Tardive dyskinesia. A clinical and therapeutic review. *Psiquiatría Biológica, 21*, 1-42.

Bena, F., Bruno, D. L., Eriksson, M., van Ravenswaaij-Arts, C., Stark, Z., Dijkhuizen, T., Schoumans, J. (2013). Molecular and clinical characterization of 25 individuals with exonic deletions of NRXN1 and comprehensive review of the literature. *American Journal of Medical Genetics. Part B, Neuropsychiatric Genetics, 162B*, 388–403.

Bergman, H., Walker, D. M., Nikolakopoulou A., Soares-Weiser K. and Adams C. E. (2017). Systematic review of interventions for treating or preventing antipsychotic-induced tardive dyskinesia. *Health Technology Assessment, 21*, 1-218.

Branchey, M. and Branchey, L. (1984). Patterns of psychotropic drug use and tardive dyskinesia. *Journal of Clinical Psychopharmacology, 4*, 41-45.

Caligiuri, M. P., Teulings, H. L., Dean, C. E. and Lohr, J. B. (2015). A Quantitative Measure of Handwriting Dysfluency for Assessing Tardive Dyskinesia. *Journal of Clinical Psychopharmacology, 35*, 168-174.

Carbon, M., Hsieh, C. H., Kane, J. M. and Correll, C. U. (2017). Tardive dyskinesia prevalence in the period of second-generation antipsychotic use: a meta-analysis. *Journal of Clinical Psychiatry, 78*, 264-278.

Carbon, M., Kane, J. M., Leucht, S. and Correll, C. U. (2018). Tardive dyskinesia risk with first and second generation antipsychotics in comparative randomized controlled trials: a meta-analysis. *World Psychiatry, 17*, 330-340.

Caroff, S. N., Mu, F., Ayyagari, R., Schilling, T., Abler, V. and Carroll, B. (2018). Hospital utilization rates following antipsychotic dose reductions: implications for tardive dyskinesia. *BMC Psychiatry, 18*, 306.

Caroff, S. N. and Campbell, E. C. (2016). Drug-induced extrapyramidal syndromes: implications for contemporary practice. P*sychiatric Clinic of North America, 39*, 391-411.

Caroff, S. N., Campbell, E. C. and Carroll, B. (2017). Pharmacological treatment of tardive dyskinesia: recent developments. *Expert Review of Neurotherapeutics, 17*, 871-881.

Castro, F. A., Carrizo, E., Rincón, D. P., Rincón, C. A., Asián, T., Medina-Leendertz, S. J. and Bonilla, E. (2011). Effectiveness of melatonin in tardive dyskinesia. *Investigación Clínica, 52*, 252-260.

Chen, C. N., Chang, K. C., Wang, M. H., Tseng, H. C. and Soung, H. S. (2018). Protective Effect of L-Theanine on Haloperidol-Induced Orofacial. *Chinese Journal of Physiology, 61*, 35-41.

Cho, C. H. and Lee, H. J. (2012). Oxidative stress and tardive dyskinesia: Pharmacogenetic evidence. *Progress in Neuro-Psychopharmacology & Biological Psychiatry, 46,* 207-13.

Citrome, L. (2017). Clinical management of tardive dyskinesia: five steps to success. *Journal Neurologic of Science, 383,* 199-204.

Cornett, E. M., Novitch, M., Kaye, A. D., Kata, V. and Kaye, A. M. (2017). Medication-induced tardive dyskinesia: a review and update. *Ochsner Journal, 17*, 162-174.

Correll, C. U. and Schenk, E. M. (2008). Tardive dyskinesia and new antipsychotics. *Current Opinion in Psychiatry, 21*, 151-156.

Correll, C. U., Rubio, J. M. and Kane, J. M. (2018). What is the risk-benefit ratio of long-term antipsychotic treatment in people with schizophrenia? *World Psychiatry, 17,* 149-160.

Correll, C. U. and Carbon, M. (2017). A new class of VMAT-2 inhibitors for tardive dyskinesia. *Lancet Psychiatry*, *4*, 574-575.

D'Abreu, A., Akbar, U. and Friedman, J. H. (2018). Tardive dyskinesia: epidemiology. *Journal of the Neurological Sciences, 389*, 17-20.

Diefenderfer, L. A., Nelson, L. A., Elliott, E., Liu, Y., Iuppa, C., Winans, E. and Sommi, R. W. (2014). Effectiveness evaluation of a pharmacist-driven monitoring database for tardive dyskinesia. *Hospital Pharmacy, 49*, 544-548.

Diehl, A., Reinhard, I., Schmitt, A., Mann, K. and Gattaz, W. F. (2009). Does the degree of smoking affect the severity of tardive dyskinesia? A longitudinal clinical trial. *European Psychiatry, 24*, 33-40.

Elkashef, A. M. and Wyatt, R. J. (1999). Tardive dyskinesia: possible involvement of free radicals and treatment with vitamin E. *Schizophrenia Bulletin, 25*, 731–740.

Emsley, R., Turner, H. J., Schronen, J., Botha, K., Smit, R. and Oosthuizen P. P. (2004). A single-blind, randomized trial comparing quetiapine and haloperidol in the treatment of tardive dyskinesia. *Journal Clinical Psychiatry, 65*, 696-701.

Faurbye, A., Rasch, P. J., Petersen, P. B., Brandborg, G. and Pakkenberg, H. (1964). Neurological symptoms in pharmacotherapy of psychosis. *Acta Psychiatrica Scandinava, 40*, 10-27.

Fedorenko, O. Y., Loonen, A. J., Lang, F., Toshchakova, V. A., Boyarko, E. G., Semke, A. V., Bokhan, N. A., Govorin, N. V., Aftanas, L. I. and Ivanova, S. A. (2015). Association study indicates a protective role of phosphatidylinositol-4-phosphate-5-kinase against tardive dyskinesia. *International Journal of Neuropsychopharmacology, 18*, 1-6.

Freedman, R., Bell, J. and Kirch, D. (1980). Clonidine therapy for coexisting psychosis and tardive dyskinesia. *Ameriacn Journal of Psychiatry, 137*, 629-30.

Frei, K., Truong, D. D., Fahn, S., Jankovic, J. and Hauser, R. (2018). The nosology of tardive syndromes. *Journal of the Neurological Sciences, 389*, 10-16.

Ganzini, I., Casey, D. E., Hoffman, W. F. and Heintz, R. T. (1992). Tardive dyskinesia and diabetes mellitus. *Psychopharmacology Bulletin, 28*, 281-286.

Gittis, A. H., Leventhal, D. K., Fensterheim, B. A., Pettibone, J. R., Berke, J. D. and Kreitzer, A. C. (2011). Selective inhibition of striatal fast-spiking interneurons causes dyskinesia. *The Journal of Neuroscience: the official journal of the Society for Neuroscience, 31*, 15727–15731.

Glazer, W. M. (2000). Expected incidence of tardive dyskinesia associated with atypical antipsychotics. *Journal of Clinical Psychiatry, 61*, 21–26.

Glazer, W. M., Morgenstern, H. and Doucette, J. T. (1993). Predicting the long-term risk of tardive dyskinesia in outpatients maintained on neuroleptic medications. *Journal of Clinical Psychiatry, 54*, 133-139.

Gunne, L., Häggström, J. and Sjöquist, B. (1984). Association with persistent neuroleptic-induced dyskinesia of regional changes in brain GABA synthesis. *Nature, 309*, 347-349.

Guy, W. (1976). ECDEU *Assessment Manual for Psychopharmacology: publication ADM,* 76-358. Washington DC: U.S. Department of Public Health, Education, and Welfare, 534-537.

Hauser, R. A., Factor, S. A., Marder, S. R., Knesevich, M. A., Ramirez, P. M., Jimenez, R., Burke, J., Liang, G. S. and O'Brien, C. F. (2017) KINECT 3: a phase 3 randomized, double-blind, placebo-controlled trial of valbenazine for tardive dyskinesia. *American Journal of Psychiatry, 174*, 476-484.

Hori, H., Ohmori, O., Shinkai, T., Kojima, H., Okano, C., Suzuki, T. and Nakamura, J. (2000). Manganese superoxide dismutase gene polymorphism and schizophrenia: relation to tardive dyskinesia. *Neuropsychopharmacology, 23*, 170-177.

Jankovic, J. (2017). An update on new and unique uses of botulinum toxin in movement disorders. *Official Journal of the International Society on Toxinology, 147*, 84-88.

Jankovic, J. and Clarence-Smith, K. (2011). Tetrabenazine for the treatment of chorea and other hyperkinetic movement disorders. *Expert Review of Neurotherapeutics, 11,* 1509-1523.

Jimenez-Shahed, J. and Jankovic, J. (2013). Tetrabenazine for treatment of chorea associated with Huntington's disease. *Expert Opinion on Orphan Drugs, 1,* 423-436.

Kane, J. M. and Smith, J. M. (1982). Tardive dyskinesia: prevalence and risk factors, 1959-1979. *Archives of General Psychiatry, 39*, 473-481.

Kane, J. M., Woerner, M. and Lieberman, J. (1988). Tardive dyskinesia: prevalence, incidence and risk factors. *Journal of Clinical Psychopharmacology, 8*, 52-56.

Kane, J., Woener, M., Weinhold, P. and Wegner, J. (1982). Results from a prospective study of tardive dyskinesia development: preliminary findings over a 2-year period. *Psychopharmacology Bulletin, 18*, 82-83.

Kenney, C. and Jankovic, J. (2006). Tetrabenazine in the treatment of hyperkinetic movement disorders. *Expert Review of Neurotherapeutics,* 6, 7-17.

Kiriakakis, V., Bhatia, K. P., Guinn, N. P. and Marsden, C. D. (1998). The natural history of tardive dystonia. A long-term follow-up study of 107 cases. *Brain, 121,* 2053-2066.

Kulkarni, S. K. and Naidu, P. S. (2003). Pathophysiology and drug therapy of tardive dyskinesia: current concepts and future perspectives. *Drugs Today, 39,* 19-49.

Lanning, R., Lett, T. A., Tiwari, A. K., Brandl, E. J., de Luca, V., Voineskos, A. N., Potkin, S. G., Lieberman, J. A., Meltzer, H. Y., Müller, D. J., Remington, G., Kennedy, J. L. and Zai, C. C. (2017). Association study between the neurexin-1 gene and tardive dyskinesia. *Human Psychopharmacology: Clinical and Experimental, 32,* e2568.

Lavania, S., Praharaj, S. M., Bains, H. S., Kumar, S., Rathore, D. M. S., Mohanty, S. and Nayak, M. (2013). Does Tardive Dysmentia Really Exist? *The Journal of Neuropsychiatry and Clinical Neurosciences, 25,* 58-62.

Lawal, O. H. and Krantz, D. E. (2013). SLC18: vesicular neurotransmitter transporters for monoamines and acetylcholine. *Molecular Aspects of Medicine, 34,* 360-372.

Lerer, B., Segman, R. H., Fangerau, H., Daly, A. K., Basile, V. S., Cavallaro, R., Aschauer, H. N., McCreadie, R. G., Ohlraun, S., Ferrier, N., Masellis, M., Verga, M., Sharfetter, J., Rietschel, M., Lovlie, R., Levy, U. H., Meltzer, H. Y., Kennedy, J. L., Steen, V. M. and Macciardi, F. (2002). Pharmacogenetics of tardive dyskinesia: combined analysis of 780 patients supports association with dopamine D3 receptor gene Ser9Gly polymorphism. *Neuropsychopharmacology, 27,* 105–119.

Lerner, P. P., Miodownik, C. and Lerner, V. (2015). Tardive dyskinesia (syndrome): Current concept and modern approaches to its management. *Psychiatry and Clinical Neurosciences, 69,* 321-334.

Lerner, V., Miodownik, C., Sheva, B., Bhidayasiri, R., Fahn, S., Weiner, W. J., Gronseth, G. S., Sullivan, K. L. and Zesiewicz, T. A. (2013). Evidence-based guideline: treatment of tardive syndromes: report of the guideline development subcommitte of the American Academy of Neurology. *Neurology, 81,* 463-469.

Lumetti, S., Ghiacci, G., Macaluso, G. M., Amore, M., Galli, C., Calciolari, E. and Manfredi, E. (2016). Tardive Dyskinesia, Oral Parafunction, and Implant-Supported Rehabilitation. *Case Reports in Dentistry* doi: 10.1155/2016/7167452.

Manteghi, A., Hojjat, S. K. and Javanbakht, A. (2009). Remission of tardive dystonia with electroconvulsive therapy. *Journal of Clinical Psychopharmacology,* 29, 314-315.

Margolese, H. C., Chouinard, G., Kolivakis, T. T., Beauclair, L., Miller, R. and Annable, L. (2005). Tardive dyskinesia in the era of typical and atypical antipsychotics. Part 1: pathophysiology and mechanisms of induction. *Canadian Journal of Psychiatry, 50,* 541–547.

Martino, D. and Morgante, F. (2017). Movement disorders and chronic psychosis *Neurology Clinical Practice, 7,* 163-169.

Mehanna, R., Hunter, C., Davidson, A., Jimenez-Shahed, J. and Jankovic, J. (2013). Analysis of CYP2D6 genotype and response to tetrabenazine. *Movement Disorders, 28,* 210-215.

Mejia, N. I. and Jankovic, J. (2010). Tardive dyskinesia and withdrawal emergent syndrome in children. *Expert Review of Neurotherapeutics, 10,* 893-901.

Meng, D. W., Liu, H. G., Yang, A. C., Zhang, K. and Zhang, J. G. (2016). Long-term effects of subthalamic nucleus deep brain stimulation in tardive dystonia. *Chinese Medical Journal, 129,* 1257-1258.

Morigaki, R., Mure, H., Kaji, R., Nagahiro, S. and Goto, S. (2016). Therapeutic perspective on tardive syndrome with special reference to deep brain stimulation. *Frontiers in Psychiatry, 7,* 207.

Niemann, N. and Jankovic, J. (2018). Treatment of tardive dyskinesia: A general overview with focus on the vesicular monoamine transporter 2 inhibitors. *Drugs, 78,* 525-541.

O'Brien, C. F., Jimenez, R., Hauser, R. A., Factor, S. A, Burke, J., Mandri, D. and Castro-Gayol, J. C. (2015). A selective monoamine transport inhibitor for the treatment of tardive dyskinesia: a randomized, double-blind, placebo-controlled study. *Movement Disorders, 30,* 1681-1687.

Ormerod, S., McDowell, S. E., Coleman, J. J. and Ferner, R. E. (2008). Ethnic differences in the risks of adverse reactions to drugs used in the treatment of psychoses and depression: a systematic review and meta-analysis. *Drug Safety, 31*, 597-607.

Pantelis, C., Stuart, G. W., Nelson, H. E., Robbins, T. W. and Barnes, T. R. E. (2001). Spatial Working Memory Deficits in Schizophrenia: Relationship with Tardive Dyskinesia and Negative Symptoms. *The American Journal of Psychiatry, 158,* 1276-1285.

Pappa, S., Tsouli, S., Apostolou, G., Mavreas, V. and Konitsiotis, S. (2010). Effects of amantadine on tardive dyskinesia: a randomized, double-blind, placebo-controlled study. *Journal of Clinical Neuropharmacology, 33*, 271-275.

Pedroso, J. L., Henriques, C. C., Escorcio, M. L., Baiense, R. F., Suarez, M. M., Dutra, L. A., Braga-Neto, P. and Povoas, O. G. (2011). Ginkgo biloba and cerebral bleeding. *Neurologist, 17,* 89-90.

Peña, M. S., Yaltho, T. C. and Jankovic, J. Tardive dyskinesia and other movement disorders secondary to aripiprazole (2011). *Movement Disorders, 26*, 147-152.

Potvin, S., Blanchet, P. and Stip, E. (2009). Substance abuse is associated with increased extrapyramidal symptoms in schizophrenia: a meta-analysis. *Schizophrenia Research, 113*, 181-188.

Rao, A. S. and Camilleri, M. (2010). Review article: metoclopramide and tardive dyskinesia. *Alimentary Pharmacology & Therapeutics, 31*, 11-19.

Reiter, R. J. and Maestroni, G. J. (1999). Melatonin in relation to the antioxidative defense and immune systems: Possible implications for cell and organ transplantation. *Journal of Molecular Medicine, 77*, 36-39.

Samad, N. (2015). Rice bran oil prevents neuroleptic-induced extrapyramidal symptoms in rats: Possible antioxidant mechanisms. *Journal of Food and Drug Analysis, 23,* 370-375.

Schrodt, G. R. Jr., Wright, J. H., Simpson, R., Moore, D. P. and Chase, S. (1982). Treatment of tardive dyskinesia with propranolol. *Journal of Clinical Psychiatry, 43*, 328-331.

Seeman, P. (2010). Dopamine D2 receptors as treatment targets in schizophrenia. *Clinical Schizophrenia & Related Psychoses, 4*, 56–73.

Segman, R. H., Heresco-Levy, U., Finkel, B., Goltser, T., Shalem, R., Schlafman, M., Dorevitch, A., Yakir, A., Greenberg, D., Lerner, A., Lerer, B. (2001). Association between the serotonin 2A receptor gene and tardive dyskinesia in chronic schizophrenia. *Molecular Psychiatry, 6*, 225–229.

Shamir, E., Barak, Y., Shalman, I., Laudon, M., Zisapel, N., Tarrasch, R. Elizur, A. and Weizman, R. (2001). Melatonin treatment for tardive dyskinesia: A double-blind, placebo-controlled, crossover study. *Archives of General* Psychiatry, *58*, 1049-1052.

Silver, J. M., Yudofsky, S. C., Kogan, M. and Katz, B. L. (1986). Elevation of thioridazine plasma levels by propranolol. *American Journal of Psychiatry, 143*, 1290-1292.

Silvestri, S., Seeman, M. V., Negrete, J. C., Houle, S., Shammi, C. M., Remington, G. J., Kapur, S., Zipursky, R. B., Wilson, A. A., Christensen, B. K. and Seeman, P. (2000). Increased dopamine D2 receptor binding after long-term treatment with antipsychotics in humans: a clinical PET study. *Psychopharmacology (Berl), 152*, 174–80.

Solmi, M., Pigato, G., Kane, J. M. and Correll, C. U. (2018). Clinical risk factors for the development of tardive dyskinesia. *Journal of the Neurological Sciences, 389*, 21-27.

Souza, R. P., Remington, G., Chowdhury, N. I., Lau, M. K., Voineskos, A. N., Lieberman, J. A., Meltzer, H. Y. and Kennedy, J. L. (2010). Association study of the GSK-3B gene with tardive dyskinesia in European Caucasians. *European Neuropsychopharmacology, 20*, 688–694.

Spindler, M. A., Galifianakis, N. B., Wilkinson, J. R. and Duda, J. E. (2013). Globus pallidus interna deep brain stimulation for tardive dyskinesia: case report and review of the literature. *Parkinsonism Related Disorders, 19*, 141-147.

Stewart, R. M., Rollins, J., Beckham, B. and Roffman, M. (1982). Baclofen in tardive dyskinesia patients maintained on neuroleptics. *Clinical Neuropharmacology, 5,* 365-373.

Tammenmaa, I. A., Sailas, E., McGrath, J. J., Soares-Weiser, K. and Wahlbeck, K. (2004). Systematic review of cholinergic drugs for neuroleptic-induced tardive dyskinesia: a meta-analysis of randomized controlled trials. *Progress in Neuro-Psychopharmacology and Biological Psychiatry, 28,* 1099-1107.

Tamminga, C. A., Thaker, G. K., Moran, M., Kakigi, T. and Gao X. M. (1994). Clozapine in tardive dyskinesia: observations from human and animal model studies. *Journal Clinical Psychiatry, 55(suppl B),* 102-106.

Tan, E. C., Chong, S. A., Mahendran, R., Dong, F. and Tan, C. H. (2001). Susceptibility to neuroleptic-induced tardive dyskinesia and the T102C polymorphism in the serotonin type 2A receptor. *Biological Psychiatry, 50,* 144–147.

Tan, E. K. and Jankovic, J. (2000). Tardive and idiopathic oromandibular dystonia: a clinical comparison. *Journal of Neurology, Neurosurgery and Psychiatry, 68,* 186-190.

Telfer, S., Shivashankar, S., Krishnadas, R., McCreadie, R. G. and Kirkpatrick, B. (2011). Tardive dyskinesia and deficit schizophrenia. *Acta Psychiatrica Scandinavica, 124,* 357-362.

Tenback, D. E. and van Harten, P. N. (2011). Epidemiology and risk factors for (tardive) dyskinesia. *International Review of Neurobiology, 98,* 211-230.

Tenback, D. E., van Harten, P. N. and van Os, J. (2009). Non-therapeutic risk factors for onset of tardive dyskinesia in schizophrenia: a meta-analysis. *Movement Disorders, 24,* 2309-2315.

Tenback, D. E., Van Harten, P. N., Sloof, C. J. and van Os, J. (2006). Evidence that early extrapyramidal symptoms predict later tardive dyskinesia: a prospective analysis of 10.000 patients in the European schizophrenia outpatient health outcomes (SOHO) study. *American Journal of Psychiatry, 163,* 1438-1440.

Teo, J. T., Edwards, M. J. and Bhatia, K. (2012). Tardive dyskinesia is caused by maladaptive synaptic plasticity: a hypothesis. *Movement Disorders, 27*, 1205-1215.

Thaker, G. K., Tamminnga, C. A., Alphs, L. D., Lafferman, J., Ferraro, T. N. and Hare, T. A. (1987). Brain gamma-aminobutyric acid abnormality in tardive dyskinesia. Reduction in cerebrospinal fluid GABA levels and therapeutic response to GABA agonist treatment. *Archives of General Psychiatry, 44*, 522-529.

Todarello, G., Feng, N., Kolachana, B. S., Li, C., Vakkalanka, R., Bertolino, A. and Straub, R. E. (2014). Incomplete penetrance of NRXN1 deletions in families with schizophrenia. *Schizophrenia Research, 155*, 1–7.

Turrone, P., Remington, G., Kapur, S. and Nobrega, J. N. (2003). The relationship between dopamine D2 receptor occupancy and the vacuous chewing movement syndrome in rats. *Psychopharmacology (Berl), 165*, 166–171.

Turrone, P., Seeman, M. V. and Silvestri, S. (2000). Estrogen receptor activation and tardive dyskinesia. *Canadian Journal of Psychiatry, 45*, 288-290.

Van Harten, P. N., Bakker, P. R., Mentzel, C. L., Tijssen, M. A. and Tenback, D. E. (2014). Movement disorders and psychosis, a complex marriage. *Frontiers in Psychiatry, 5*, 190.

Vasan, S. and Padhy, R. K. (2019). Tardive Dyskinesia. *StatPearls - NCBI Bookshelf.*

Venegas, P., Millán, M. and Miranda, M. (2003). Tardive dyskinesia. *Revista Chilena de Neuropsiquiatría, 41*, 131-138.

Vijayakumar, D. and Jankovic, J. (2016). Drug-induced dyskinesia, part 2: Treatment of tardive dyskinesia. *Drugs, 76*, 779-787.

Vinuela, A. and Kang, U. J. (2014). Reversibility of Tardive Dyskinesia Syndrome. *Tremor and Other Hyperkinetic Movements, 4*, 282.

Waln, O. and Jankovic, J. (2013). An update on tardive dyskinesia: from phenomenology to treatment. *Tremor and Other Hyperkinetic Movements 3*, 1-11.

Wolf, M. A., Yassa, R. and Llorca, P. M. (1993). Neuroleptic-induced movement disorders: historical perspectives. *Encephale, 19*, 657–661.

Wu, J. Q., Chen, D. C., Xiu, M. H., Tan, Y. L., Yang, F. D., Kosten, T. R. and Zhang, X. Y. (2013). Tardive dyskinesia is associated with greater cognitive impairment in schizophrenia. *Progress in Neuro-Psychopharmacology and Biological Psychiatry, 46,* 71-77.

Yanan, H., Lizhen, P., Fei, T., Geying, W., Chenhu, L. and Lingjing, J. (2017). A Cross-Sectional Study on the Characteristics of Tardive Dyskinesia in Patients with Chronic Schizophrenia. *Shanghai Archives of Psychiatry, 29,* 295-303.

Yasui-Furukori, N., Nakamura, K., Katagai, H. and Kaneko, S. (2014). The effects of electroconvulsive therapy on tardive dystonia or dyskinesia induced by psychotropic medication: a retrospective study. (2014). *Neuropsychiatric Disease and Treatment, 10,* 1209-1212.

Zhang, W. F., Tan, Y. L., Zhang, X. Y., Chan, R. C., Wu, H. R. and Zhou, D. F. (2011). Extract of Ginkgo biloba treatment for tardive dyskinesia in schizophrenia: a randomized, double-blind, placebo-controlled trial. *Journal Clinical Psychiatry, 72,* 615-621.

Zhang, Z. J., Zhang, X. B., Hou, G., Yao, H. and Reynolds, G. P. (2003). Interaction between polymorphisms of the dopamine D3 receptor and manganese superoxide dismutase genes in susceptibility to tardive dyskinesia. *Psychiatry Genetics, 13,* 187–192.

In: Understanding Dyskinesia
Editor: Jan Dvořák
ISBN: 978-1-53618-502-7
© 2020 Nova Science Publishers, Inc.

Chapter 3

PHYSICAL ACTIVITY, EXERCISE AND DYSKINESIA

Ana Elisa Speck[1,], Rui Daniel Schroder Prediger[1] and Aderbal Silva Aguiar Junior[2]*

[1]Experimental Laboratory of Neurodegenerative Diseases, Department of Pharmacology, Federal University of Santa Catarina (UFSC), Florianópolis, SC, Brazil

[2]Lab Biology of Exercise, Department of Health Sciences, Federal University of Santa Catarina (UFSC), Araranguá, SC, Brazil.

ABSTRACT

Dyskinesia is hyperkinetic abnormal involuntary movement (AIM) which includes isolated or combined chorea, dystonia, athetosis, and ballism. AIM can be found in some disorders, such as Levodopa-induced dyskinesia (LIDs) in Parkinson's disease, tardive dyskinesia in schizophrenia, and paroxysmal dyskinesia. The purpose of this chapter is to review the acute effects of physical activity and exercise adaptation (eg rehabilitation) on different types of dyskinesia. Physical activity showed antidyskinetic effects in Parkinson's LIDs, with well-defined biological mechanisms. Acute exercise does not modify abnormal respiratory patters in schizophrenia. These patients have a normal response to progressive exercise and inspiratory time. Sustained walking or running may induce paroxysmal dyskinesia in healthy subjects. We will deeply explore this evidence.

Keywords: dyskinesia, physical exercise, Levodopa-induced dyskinesia, tardive dyskinesia and paroxysmal dyskinesia

INTRODUCTION

Dyskinesia occurs in various medical conditions and is the term used to describe unintentional, involuntary, and uncontrollable movements. This includes spasms, twists, or simple restlessness (Fahn 2000; Del-Bel et al. 2015). Dyskinesia should not be confused with tics that are sudden, repetitive, non-rhythmic movements involving isolated muscle groups, for example, blinking or clearing the throat. It can affect each person differently, both in timing and frequency and severity. It may or may not interfere considerably with a patient's daily life activities or it may be light and almost imperceptible. Generally speaking, the movements are fast as a dance, known as chorea. At times the movements are known as dystonia, which causes sustained involuntary muscle spasms and contractions. Dystonia is slower, painful and contorted, forcing the body into unnatural postures. At times the choreic movements and dystonias overlap and you can try them at the same time.

This type abnormal involuntary movement (AIM) is very common in Parkinson's disease (PD) and may result from the disease process itself or as a side-effect of levodopa medication used to treat symptoms. Dyskinesia may be present when drugs have worn off, such as first thing in the morning ('off'-medication dyskinesia) or during the day when the medication is working ('on'-medication dyskinesia). The most common types of dyskinesia in Parkinson's disease are chorea, ballism, dystonia and myoclonus. Although these movement disorders are problematic, many individuals would rather be on dyskinesia rather than off without dyskinesia. When levodopa reaches its peak of effectiveness and dopamine levels are at their highest, "maximum dose dyskinesia" may occur. On the other hand, and less commonly, dyskinesia can also occur when levodopa is just beginning to take effect or when it is running out. This is known as "dysphasic dyskinesia." Different parts of the body may be affected, but the most common areas are the limbs and trunk.

Dyskinesia can occurs also in ideopathically in antipsychotic-naïve patients with psychotic disorders, drug induced (antipsychotics or other drugs), in hereditary diseases, in a systemic or neurological disease, or as a result of psychological stress. Spontaneous hyperkinetic dyskinesia such as "grimacing" and "irregular movements of tongue and lips" are prevalent in antipsychotic-naïve psychotic patients: Kraepelin and Bleuler described the phenomenon more than 100 years ago (Koning et al. 2010). In this case is known as tardive dyskinesia (TD) is a syndrome that subsumes a variety of iatrogenic movement disorders. There are also some other established risk factors for developing TD that are not drug-related. Age seems consistently associated with the development, persistence, and progression of TD. Women appear to be at increased risk for TD (Haro and Salvador-Carulla 2006). Moreover, spontaneous dyskinesia in medication-naïve patients with schizophrenia and rarely, in the general population, were reported (Lerner and Miodownik 2011; Merrill, Lyon, and Matiaco 2013). The defining characteristics of TD include its delayed onset—hence the name "tardive"— signifying a delay of weeks to months until symptoms appear, and dyskinetic (abnormal, involuntary) movements. Depending on the severity, tardive dyskinesia can have a quite adverse functional impact that can be debilitating, stigmatizing, and associated with increased mortality.

Paroxysmal dyskinesias (PxDs) are a relatively rare subset of hyperkinetic movement disorders that are defined by their episodic nature. Patients present with repeated episodes of dyskinesia (dystonia, chorea, or both) that have sudden onset and, after a duration that ranges from seconds to days, remit entirely and subsequently recur in a stereotyped fashion. They may be primary or secondary, and when primary they are often associated with genetic causes. Paroxysmal kinesigenic dyskinesia (PKD) is triggered by sudden movements, paroxysmal exercise-induced dyskinesia (PED) is triggered by sustained physical effort, and paroxysmal nonkinesigenic dyskinesia (PNKD) is not triggered by movement, but sometimes is provoked by consumption of coffee or alcohol or by stress. (Demirkiran and Jankovic 1995) Many of the PxDs can be co-morbid with other neurological disorders that are suggestive of an underlying channelopathy[1], such as epilepsy and migraine.

Physical exercise can modify different types of dyskinesias in different ways. In this chapter, we will identify the most varied types of dyskinesias and the relationship with exercise and physical activity in clinical studies and dyskinetic animal models. However, many studies, despite strong evidence on the benefits of exercise in various forms in L-DOPA-induced dyskinesia (LIDs), but not in relation to TD and PED. However, the main role of physical therapy and exercise in dyskinesia: palliative, curative or neuroprotective? This chapter attempts to review the evidence reported in different clinical studies and animal models to provide a comprehensive picture of the role of physical therapy and exercise.

L-DOPA INDUCED DYSKINESIA AND EXERCISE

The treatment of PD is very complex due to the progression of the disease and a set of motor and non-motor signs and engines combined with early and late side effects associated with therapeutic interventions. Although there are no approved neuroprotective treatments to slow the progression of disease, some pharmacological palliative therapies are available, as well as surgical alternatives and other approaches such as physical exercise and physiotherapy.

Since the neurotransmitter DA does not cross the barrier hematopoietic the administration of its precursor L-DOPA consists of the main pharmacological strategy to re-establish, less temporarily, dopaminergic neurotransmission and relieving the motor symptoms of the patients (Calne

---

[1] Channelopathies are a heterogeneous group of disorders resulting from the dysfunction of ion channels located in the membranes of all cells and many cellular organelles. These include diseases of the nervous system (e.g., generalized epilepsy with febrile seizures plus, familial hemiplegic migraine, episodic ataxia, and hyperkalemic and hypokalemic periodic paralysis).

1993; Horstink et al. 2006; Kieburtz 2006). The clinical use of L-DOPA in PD started of the 1960s, and remains to this day as the most effective therapy to attenuate PD cardinal motor symptoms (Fox et al. 2011). Motor dysfunctions in are the main target of pharmacological treatment, with L-3,4-dihydroxyphenylalanine (L-DOPA) being the most effective drug (Jenner 2008). The primary complication of L-DOPA therapy is the development of dyskinesia and motor fluctuations; thus, objective of current physical exercise research is to prolong the antiparkinsonian effects of L-DOPA to improve patients's quality of life.

However, there exists a broad list of pharmacological agents which include: inhibitors of L-aromatic amino acid decarboxylase enzyme, monoamine oxidase inhibitors, catechol-O-methyl transferase inhibitors, dopaminergic agonists and anticholinergic drugs. Other non-pharmacological strategies that are taken into account include cell transplant therapy and deep brain stimulation (DBS) (Kaminer, Thakur, and Evinger 2015). More recently, another terapy and to PD is continuous administration of levodopa-carbidopa intestinal gel (LCIG), that reduces variability in levodopa plasma levels and improves motor complications associated with chronic oral levodopa treatment (Wang, Li, and Chen 2018). Previously published data have demonstrated that LCIG therapy not only reduces "Off" time and dyskinesia, but also improves a patient's ability to perform activities of daily living (ADL), treat his or her nonmotor symptoms (Standaert et al. 2017) and improve their quality of life.

However, despite all pharmacological strategies, the use of L-DOPA remains the most effective treatment for the motor symptoms of these patients. Thus; it becomes relevant to study the interactions between the L-DOPA and the physical exercise, can modulate the dopaminergic neurotransmission. For example, in animal models, running exercise for three weeks increases the synthesis and the release of DA in DP in C57BL/6 mice model of PD treated with a low dose of L-DOPA (5 mg/kg) (Archer and Fredriksson 2010; Fredriksson et al. 2011). In addition, the physical exercise may increase the mRNA levels of the receptors dopaminergic neurons of the D2 type in dopaminergic neurons in the striatum after treadmill exercise for 30 days in mice treated with MPTP (Fisher et al.

2004). Another study using neuroimaging in mice treated with MPTP and exposed during 6 weeks on treadmill exercise showed an increase in expression of striatal D2 receptors in exercised animals (Vuckovic et al. 2010). These adaptations in neurotransmission exercise-induced dopaminergic reactions may be involved.

Exercise can be have an antidyskinetic effect in clinical trials showing a decrease in the dyskinesia in patients with PD after intensive rehabilitation treatment (2 times a day) during 4 weeks, 5 days per week (Frazzitta, Bertotti, et al. 2012) (Figure 1). The rehabilitation protocol (which consisted of gait training exercises, treadmill training) resulted in a 71% reduction in the dyskinesia, whereas the patients who performed the rehabilitation did not (only once a day) had a more modest reduction (only 8%) in the LIDs score. This same group showed in a study with duration of 6 months that this intense rehabilitation protocol improvement of the dyskinesia score, as well as, the UPDRS scale, and reduction the L-DOPA dosage during the 6 months after treatment (Frazzitta, Morelli, et al. 2012).

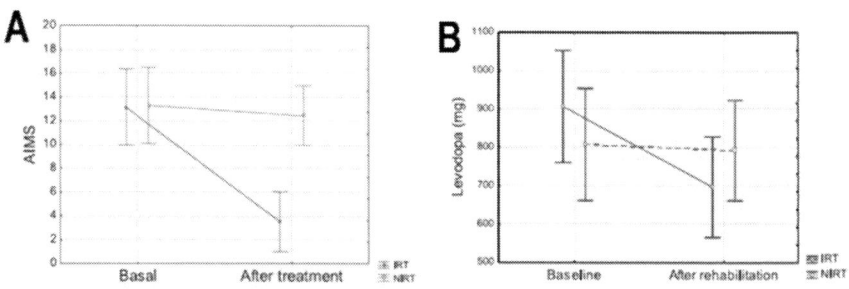

Figure 1. Graphical representation time-treatment interaction for the variable AIMS. Differences in treatment effect are reflected by differences in the slope of the lines joining the mean value AIMS at baseline and after rehabilitation in the two groups (A). The patients that make an IRT protocol could be decrease a levodopa dosage after rehabilitation protocol (B) AIMS - Abnormal involuntary movement scale; IRT - Intensive rehabilitation treatment; NIRT - non-intensive rehabilitation treatment.

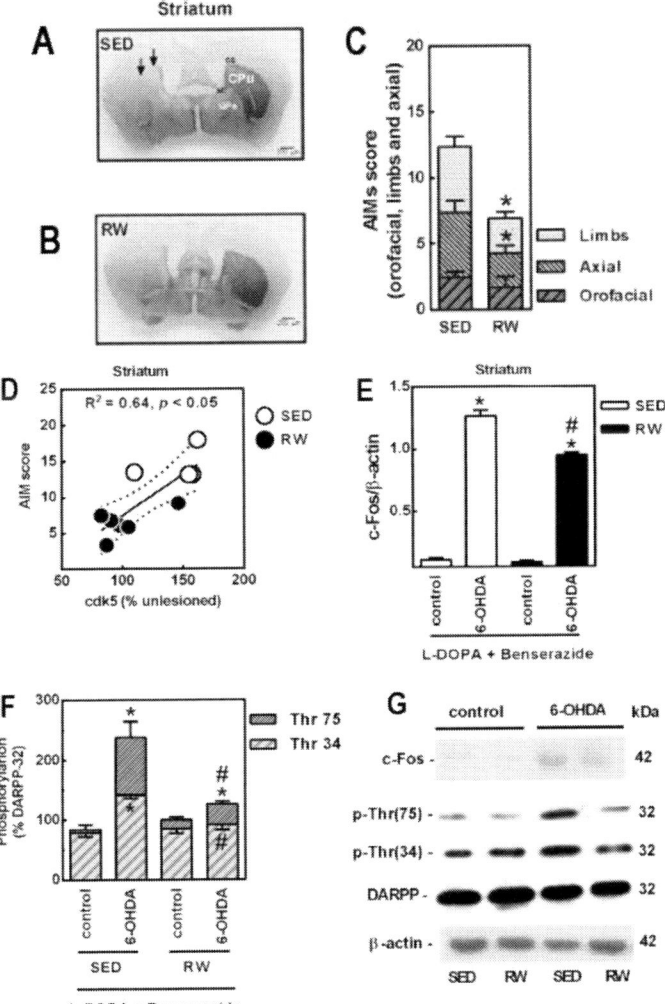

Figure 2. Exercise and L-DOPA/benserazide (25/12.5 mg/kg, i.p.) showed no effect on neurodegeneration, evaluated as a decreased immunoreactivity of tyrosine hydroxylase in the lesioned striatum (A, B). However, exercise was effective in reducing LIDs (C). The severity of L-DOPA-induced dyskinesia correlated with increased striatal levels of cdk5 (D) and c-Fos (E). L-DOPA also triggered a hyperphosphorylation of DARPP-32 at Thr(34) and Thr(75) sites in sedentary mice (F). Notably, exercise (RW) decreased these neurochemical changes typically associated with L-DOPA-induced dyskinesia. AIM, abnormal involuntary movements; cdk5, CPu, Caudate-putamen; GPe, external globus pallidus; cyclin-dependent kinase 5; DARPP-32, dopamine and cAMP-regulated phosphoprotein 32 kDa; RW, running wheel; SED, sedentary; st, stria terminalis; Thr, threonine residue; 6-OHDA, 6-hydroxydopamine.

The first work that showed the potential antidiskinetic effect of physical exercise on LIDs in mice was puplish in 2013 by Aguiar et al. (Aguiar et al. 2013). This work the C57BL/6 mice were submitted to unilateral lesion with 6-OHDA (12 µg), after they received a L-DOPA plus benzerazide. At the same time they did exercise. In this study, animals injured with 6-OHDA were trained in running wheel (voluntary exercise) during 14 days together with the daily treatment of the L-DOPA association (25 mg/kg, i.p.) + benserazide (12.5 mg/kg). After the protocol training, it was possible to observe that there was no modification of the lesion caused by 6-OHDA (Figure 2-A). Physical exercise decreased axial and limb dyskinesia, but not orofacial (Figure 2 C). Moreover, in this same work, the antidiskinetic effects of voluntary exercise were associated with normalization of dopaminergic signaling in the striatum, specifically, hyperphosphorylation of DARPP-32 (regulated by 32 kDa phosphoprotein protein DA and cAMP), CDK5 and expression of c-Fos (Figure 2 D-G).

Additionally, after treadmill trainning in L-DOPA induced dyskinesia Swiss mice model have am antidiscnetic effect and increases striatal glial cell-derived neurotrophic factor (GDNF), levels that provide a new mechanistic view (Figure 3). Additonally, Cohen, 2003 (Cohen et al. 2003) demonstrated that the physical exercise of limb pre-injury can prevent behavioral deficits and neurochemicals induced by the administration of 6-OHDA, and related this protection from physical exercise to the increase in GDNF striatal lesions. Evidence from both in vivo and in vitro studies indicates the protective and regenerative potential of GDNF on dopaminergic neurons (d'Anglemont de Tassigny, Pascual, and Lopez-Barneo 2015). Intra-striatal pretreatment with GDNF (100 µg) during 4 weeks before 6-OHDA model was able to prevent degeneration of dopaminergic neurons (Aoi et al. 2000). In addition, the GDNF i.c.v. after injury by 6-OHDA (28 µg) restores striatal TH levels dorsolateral movement of rats, as well as improving motor symptoms animals (Kirik et al. 2001). Another great relevance, the intra-striatal GDNF injection (5 µg) reduced LIDs in MPTP-treated monkeys (Iravani et al. 2001). Taken together, these results indicate that the increase in of GDNF in the striatum of dyskinetic animals may represent an important mechanism of the modulating effect of treadmill exercise in LIDs. In this way, there are convergent evidence from clinical and experimental studies that the exercise may act as a modifying agent of PD (Aguiar Jr. et al. 2009; Mantri et al. 2018; Muller and Muhlack 2010; Toy et al. 2014) and have antidyskinetic effetcts (Aguiar et al. 2013; Frazzitta, Morelli, et al. 2012; Frazzitta, Bertotti, et al. 2012; Speck et al. 2018).

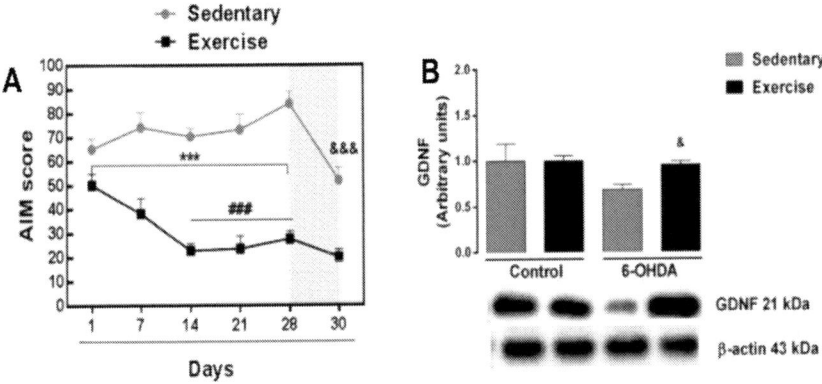

Figure 3. Exercise (treadmill) or sedentary groups, and both groups were treated with L-DOPA/benserazide (50/25 mg/kg, i.p.) during 4 weeks. Exercised mice showed a reduced AIM score from 14th, 21th, and 28th days of treatment (***$P < 0.001$ vs. sedentary; ###$P < 0.001$ vs. exercised on 1st day (A). Exercise increased the GDNF immunocontent in 6-OHDAlesioned striatum of dyskinetic mice (B).

TARDIVE DYSKINESIA AND EXERCISE

Movement disorders that may today be referred to as antipsychotic-induced tardive dyskinesia (TD), that were first observed in some patients taking antipsychotics in the 1950s and were called neuroleptic-induced parkinsonism. Such movements were acute and short lived in some cases and chronic in others. These movement disorders were eventually referred to using the term extrapyramidal side effects. The first cases of involuntary and persistent abnormal movements associated with antipsychotics were reported by Schonecker (SCHONECKER 1957) in 1957 as persistent perioral movements occurring with the use of multiple antipsychotic medications. The term tardive dyskinesia was introduced by Faurbye in 1964 (Faurbye et al. 1964), highlighting the delayed onset of the condition (Waddington 1990; Wolf, Yassa, and Llorca 1993). During the 1960s, involuntary movements that developed or worsened after the discontinuation of an antipsychotic or a reduction of its dose were also termed TD.

The definitive cause of TD is still uncertain and likely multifactorial. However, modern technology involving animal studies and data on receptor occupancy has broadened our understanding of the neurobiology underlying TD. Different hypotheses explaining the pathophysiology of TD include an upregulation of D2 and D3 receptors, dysregulated dopamine influence on the substantia nigra, striatal neurodegeneration, changes in synaptic plasticity due to surges of γ-aminobutyric acid in the striatal neurons responsible for motor coordination, oxidative trauma, and changes in 5-HT2 receptor signaling (Tarsy, Lungu, and Baldessarini 2011; Tarsy and Baldessarini 2006; Kim, Macmaster, and Schwartz 2014; Mahmoudi, Levesque, and Blanchet 2014).

The most broadly accepted explanation for TD is that chronic and substantial D2 receptor blockade causes a compensatory increase in D2 receptor synthesis (generally referred to as upregulation), which in turn leads to supersensitivity at those receptors. Researchers have observed rats developing spontaneous perioral movements as a result of long-term D2 receptor blockade from chronic administration of high doses of D2 selective drugs (ie, with high D2 receptor occupancy) and have suggested that this animal model resembles the mechanisms underlying the pathophysiology of TD in humans (Waddington 1990, 1989; Ellison and See 1989). Parsons et al. (Parsons et al. 1995) showed that rodents exposed to haloperidol had 24% and 33% increased density of striatal D2 and adenosine A2a receptors, respectively. Ginovart et al. (Ginovart et al. 2009) also found that continuous blockade of D2 receptors with haloperidol in cats led to the increased postsynaptic expression of striatal D2 receptors and suggested that this increased postsynaptic expression represents the pathophysiology of TD. In a study published in 2000, Silvestri at al (Silvestri et al. 2000) first demonstrated increased postsynaptic expression of D2 receptors in living humans using positron emission tomography, which demonstrates how advances in neuroimaging can broaden our understanding of classic concepts in neuroscience.

Few studies talk about efetcts of exercise in patients with TD. A 25-year-old woman with severe TD due to neuroleptics had substantial improvement of movements while inline skating. She received pallidal deep brain stimulation (DBS), and gait and inline skating were assessed before and after DBS; her twin sister served as a control. The authors conclude that possible explanations for her improvement include (1) balance stability required by inline skating provides external cues that are less prominent during gait; and (2) dystonia consistently responds to geste antagoniste. Since TD has variable response to treatments, the propose research into alleviating factors in TD that may advance treatment and rehabilitation in this incapacitating disorder (Casagrande et al. 2017).

The pattern ("topograpy") of dyskinesia is important for differentiating its functional impact. Truncal TD, for example, impacts gait and posture and may also exert its detrimental impact quite broadly by interfering with the ADLs that require standing or moving, such as grooming, dressing, toileting, bathing, ambulating, and transport. In contrast, orofacial TD would not have a significant impact on these tasks but would perhaps affect speech, which is required for effective interpersonal interactions or getting and keeping a job. The potential differential functional impact on motor system performance related to the topography of TD has never been determined (Strassnig, Rosenfeld, and Harvey 2018). The physical capacity of people with varied TD topography has not been examined. However it is known, that people with persistent mental illness have reduced physical capacity, at times to the point of interfering with their ADLs (Strassnig, Brar, and Ganguli 2011).

Broad-based gait, spastic gait, pelvic gyration, difficulty standing, abnormal arm swing, manneristic gait, dancing, and duck-like gait in addition to other features of TD was observed, (Kuo and Jankovic 2008) with prevalence estimates ranging from 27 to 59% of those affected with TD (Simpson and Shrivastava 1978; Yassa 1989; Lauterbach et al. 1990). Gait speed, cadence, step length, posture, arm swing, gait initiation, turning, and gait efficiency can all be impaired with TD, and such secondary impairments as limited joint range of motion, loss of lower extremity power/strength, or lack of endurance may ensue, further worsening the performance on gait-related everyday activities. Moreover, severe gait abnormalities may pose a fall risk, with associated morbidity and mortality. Gait can be comprehensively assessed in several ways, including 3D motion detectors combined with electromyography, or a gait analysis walkway that allows for temporospatial gait analysis. The interrelationship between gait and cognition suggests that gait assessments can provide a window into an understanding of the influence of cognitive function on motor performance under a cognitive load, using dual-task gait assessments (e.g., walking while performing an attention-demanding task) (Montero-Odasso et al. 2012).

Falls are a major cause of morbidity among older adults, especially for those with cognitive problems. For instance, older adults with moderate to severe cognitive impairment have a higher risk of falls, with an annual incidence of around 60–80%; twice the rate in cognitively normal older adults (Tinetti, Speechley, and Ginter 1988). The consequences of falls in the population of demented older adults are very serious; fallers with cognitive problems are approximately five times more likely to be admitted to institutional care than people with cognitive issues who do not fall (Morris et al. 1987). They are also at high risk of major fall-related injuries such as fractures and head injuries that increase mortality risk. In addition to indirect costs and caregiver burden, the direct costs of emergency, acute, rehabilitation and long-term care are substantial and increasingly unsustainable for the healthcare system.

Several forms of hyperkinetic movement disorders were described in patients with TD, including tardive stereotypy, tardive dystonia, and tardive akathisia (Stacy, Cardoso, and Jankovic 1993). Less commonly, chorea, tics, myoclonus, and tremor can also be part of the spectrum of TD (Yassa and Jones 1985). Though many patients might not be aware of their TD, it can cause complications including respiratory distress, dysphagia, dysarthria, falling, and suicide (Yassa and Jones 1985). Therefore, it is very important for clinicians to recognize the broad spectrum of phenomenology associated with TD. We describe three cases with TD and abnormal gait, which we term "tardive gait" because it is associated with onset of other features of TD.

One patient displayed dancing gait whereas the other two patients had a "duck-like" gait. Simpson and Shrivastava (Simpson and Shrivastava 1978) studied moderate to severe TD patients.

Cognitive remediation interventions were used to improve attention and executive function as well as memory in older adults without dementia. Recent studies that have specifically evaluated the effects of interventions to improve cognition on gait and fall risk. Verghese et al. (Verghese et al. 2010) conducted a pilot study in 24 older adults who were randomly assigned to either a computerized cognitive remediation intervention or a wait list. The ten participants who completed the cognitive remediation showed improvement on gait velocity during normal walking and walking while talking (dual-task) compared to baseline. While the initial findings of this pilot trial need confirmation in larger scale trials, they indicate that a non-pharmacological cognitive intervention can positively modify gait performance, especially during dual-task testing (Montero-Odasso et al. 2012).

In animal models of TD low to moderate physical exercise plays an important role in improving motor and cognitive impairments associated to monoaminergic depletion. In this work, the training exercise program consisting of 4 consecutive weeks on the running well or the treadmill attenuated the motor disruption induced by a high reserpine dose (5.0 mg/kg, s.c.) in rats (Aguiar Jr. et al. 2009).

TD-related impairments may compound physical capacity limitations. Patients with schizophrenia are two to three times more likely to have a higher mortality rate and a reduced lifespan expectancy of 13–30 years. This also applies in countries where the quality of the medical care system is generally considered to be good. Sixty percent of mortality is due to complications of metabolic and cardiovascular diseases. Weight gain applies to 72% of patients taking APs, whereas 42–60% of these patients are obese. Metabolic syndrome affects 19.4–68% of patients treated for schizophrenia (differences depend on the country, gender, age, ancestry, and medication). The risk of developing type 2 diabetes, one of the components of MS, is estimated to be two to three times higher than in the general population and nearly half of patients remain untreated (DE Hert et al. 2011).

A higher risk of cardiovascular complications is commonly related to a high frequency of diabetes, hypertension, smoking, poor nutrition, obesity, impaired lipid profile, and low physical activity (Stubbs et al. 2016, 2017), but also with the use of antipsychotics. The treatments with antipsychotics, particularly the second generation, largely contribute to metabolic complications.

Studies implemented nonpharmacological interventions such as physical activity, dietary modification, or psychoeducation that targeted physical health aspects of metabolic and physical fitness. There are many works that showed a modest but significant weight loss or improved cardiovascular fitness among patients with schizophrenia. Seven programs that implemented walking as a main intervention showed statistically significant changes in the tested parameters (Methapatara and Srisurapanont 2011; Browne et al. 2016; Wu et al. 2015; Hjorth et al. 2017). In most of them, improvement in cardiovascular fitness was achieved, and there was also a reduction in weight.

Patients with TD can be developed respiratory dysrhythmias (RDs). They are irregular respiratory rate and rhythm in association with involuntary grunts and gasping sounds (Wilcox et al. 1994). Some works described the effect of exercise and sleep on these RDs (Wilcox et al. 1994). A cycle ergometer exercise test was performed in this work, to the patient's symptom-limited maximal work load.'" Breathing frequency, minute ventilation, oxygen uptake (Vo1), and carbon dioxide production were determined on a breath-by-breath basis. The authors recorded heart rate (modified V2 and arterial oxygen saturation was monitored continuously with a pulse oximeter. In this study the paitents were compared with data derived from normal control subjects. Exertional dyspnea is a common presenting symptom of patients with RDs. The authors suggest that RDs are not the cause of premature termination of exercise in patients with TD. Maximal predicted ventilation was·only approached by one of the seven patients studied, indicating some degree of ventilatory reserve in the majority of patients. Volume and breathing frequency both increased in a normal curvilinear pattern and no patient demonstrated significant arterial oxygen desaturation during exercise.

PAROXYSMAL DYSKNESIAS AND EXERCISE

In 1740, Mount and Reback introduced the term "familial paroxysmal choreoathetosis" when they described a 23-year-old man with an autosomal dominant disorder manifested by attacks of choreoathetoid movements involving arms and legs (Zukerman, Vilanova, and Serafico 1983). The attacks occurred two to three times a day, lasted 5 minutes to hours, and were precipitated by alcohol, coffee, tea, fatigue, and smoking. Numerous reports of patients with episodic dyskinesia have followed, and several classifications were proposed to categorize this movement disorder (Lance 1977) . In 1977, Lance reviewed 100 cases reported in the literature up to that time, and added 12 patients with "familial paroxysmal dystonic choreoathetosis" (Lance 1977). He classified the cases, primarily according to the duration, as (1) paroxysmal dystonic choreoathetosis or PDC (prolonged attacks lasting 2 minutes to 4 hours), (2) paroxysmal kinesigenic choreoathetosis or PKC (brief attacks lasting seconds to 5 minutes and induced by sudden voluntary movement), and (3) intermediate form (attacks lasting 5 to 30 minutes and induced by continued exertion).

This classification, however, is problematic because it links limited scope of phenomenology to the duration of attacks. It assumes that all prolonged attacks are nonkinesigenic, and that they are manifested by dystonia or choreo athetosis, and that all brief attacks are kinesigenic and choreoathetotic. The classification offered by Goodenough and co-workers (Goodenough et al. 1978) based chiefly on etiology, categorizes the paroxysmal dyskinesia into two groups, familial and acquired. The familial cases are divided into kinesigenic (choreoathetotic, dystonic, mixed, and tonic, lasting less than 5 minutes) and nonkinesigenic (choreoathetotic and tonic, lasting more than 5 minutes) types. This classification has limitations similar to those of Lance's classification and, in addition, it fails to include sporadic (nonfamilial) and exertion-induced types of paroxysmal dyskinesia.

Paroxysmal dyskinesias (PxDs) are characterized by transient abnormal, involuntary movement, such as choreoathetosis and dystonia, but unlike the epilepsies they do not evolve into tonic–clonic seizures, and are not associated with epileptiform discharges and alterations in consciousness (Berkovic 2000). Broadly, the PxDs can be subdivided into four subgroups based upon precipitating factors: paroxysmal kinesigenic dyskinesia (PKD), paroxysmal non-kinesigenic dyskinesia (PNKD), paroxysmal exercise-induced dyskinesia (PED) and paroxysmal hypnogenic dyskinesia (PHD). The association PxDs and other neurological disorders, like epilepsy or ataxia, has occasionally been observed within one individual or family.

Interestingly, unlike LIDs, exercise in patients with this condition can activate dyskinesias. PED is characterized by attacks of dystonia and/or chorea triggered by prolonged exercise, typically lasting for 5 to 30 min (Meneret and Roze 2016). The attacks often start in the body part involved by exercise. The frequency of attacks is variable, depending on the routine level of physical exercise. The frequency of attacks varies and depends on the amount of physical PED may be accompanied by migraine without aura (Munchau et al. 2000) or a combination of alternating hemiplegic, epilepsy, and ataxia (Neville, Besag, and Marsden 1998). A combination with rolandic epilepsy and writer's cramp (RE-PED-WC) has also been reported (Guerrini et al. 1999). In some patients, PED may be the presenting sign of young-onset idiopathic Parkinson's disease, (Bozi and Bhatia 2003) for example, because of the Parkin gene.

Symptomatic treatment with antiepileptic, levodopa or acetazolamide is sometimes effective, but usually disappointing (Bhatia 2011). Specific treatment of an underlying disorder may be beneficial. Mutations in SLC2A1 are the main cause of PED, which can be isolated or part of a more complex phenotype (Weber et al. 2011; Zorzi et al. 2008; Bovi et al. 2011). Mutations in GCH1, PARK2 (encoding parkin) or other genes involved in recessive juvenile Parkinson's disease can occasionally cause PED (Dale et al. 2010). Rare genetic causes include mutations in PRRT2 (Liu et al. 2012), ATP1A3 (Roubergue et al. 2013), ADCY5 (Friedman et al. 2016), PDHA1 and PDHX (pyruvate dehydrogenase deficiency) (Barnerias et al. 2010).

CONCLUSION

The findings reviewed in this chapter indicate that exercise improves LIDs and motor impairments of PD patients and animal models. The antidyskinetic effects of voluntary or treadmill exercise were associated with normalization of dopaminergic signaling in the striatum as well as increased neurotrophic factors. Although patients with TD present a similar pattern to those affected by LIDs, there are few studies on physical exercise, especially because they are patients with mental problems. However, studies show the effects of physical exercise on dystonia and balance, cognition and cardiorespiratory capacity. And lastly PxDs is totally different pattern from the previous ones regarding the physical exercise. This condition turn presents a worsening of symptoms after the performance of a physical activity.

REFERENCES

Aguiar, A S, E L G Moreira, A A Hoeller, P A Oliveira, F M Córdova, V Glaser, R Walz, et al. 2013. "Exercise Attenuates Levodopa-Induced Dyskinesia in 6-Hydroxydopamine-Lesioned Mice." *Neuroscience* 243: 46–53. https://doi.org/10.1016/j.neuroscience.2013.03.039.

Aguiar Jr, A S, A L Araújo, T R da-Cunha, A E Speck, Z M Ignácio, N De-Mello, and R D S Prediger. 2009. "Physical Exercise Improves Motor and Short-Term Social Memory Deficits in Reserpinized Rats." *Brain Research Bulletin* 79 (6). https://doi.org/10.1016/j.brainresbull.2009.05.005.

Aoi, M, I Date, S Tomita, and T Ohmoto. 2000. "The Effect of Intrastriatal Single Injection of GDNF on the Nigrostriatal Dopaminergic System in Hemiparkinsonian Rats: Behavioral and Histological Studies Using Two Different Dosages." *Neuroscience Research* 36 (4): 319–25.

Archer, Trevor, and Anders Fredriksson. 2010. "Physical Exercise Attenuates MPTP-Induced Deficits in Mice." *Neurotoxicity Research* 18 (3–4): 313–27. https://doi.org/10.1007/s12640-010-9168-0.

Barnerias, Christine, Jean-Marie Saudubray, Guy Touati, Pascale De Lonlay, Olivier Dulac, Gerard Ponsot, Cecile Marsac, Michele Brivet, and Isabelle Desguerre. 2010. "Pyruvate Dehydrogenase Complex Deficiency: Four Neurological Phenotypes with Differing Pathogenesis." *Developmental Medicine and Child Neurology* 52 (2): e1-9. https://doi.org/10.1111/j.1469-8749.2009.03541.x.

Berkovic, S F. 2000. "Paroxysmal Movement Disorders and Epilepsy: Links across the Channel." *Neurology*. United States. https://doi.org/10.1212/wnl.55.2.169.

Bhatia, Kailash P. 2011. "Paroxysmal Dyskinesias." *Movement Disorders : Official Journal of the Movement Disorder Society* 26 (6): 1157–65. https://doi.org/10.1002/mds.23765.

Bovi, Tommaso, Alfonso Fasano, Ina Juergenson, Cinzia Gellera, Barbara Castellotti, Elena Fontana, and Michele Tinazzi. 2011. "Paroxysmal Exercise-Induced Dyskinesia with Self-Limiting Partial Epilepsy: A Novel GLUT-1 Mutation with Benign Phenotype." *Parkinsonism & Related Disorders* 17 (6): 479–81. https://doi.org/10.1016/j.parkreldis.2011.03.015.

Bozi, Maria, and Kailash P Bhatia. 2003. "Paroxysmal Exercise-Induced Dystonia as a Presenting Feature of Young-Onset Parkinson's Disease." *Movement Disorders : Official Journal of the Movement Disorder Society* 18 (12): 1545–47. https://doi.org/10.1002/mds.10597.

Browne, Julia, David L Penn, Claudio L Battaglini, and Kelsey Ludwig. 2016. "Work out by Walking: A Pilot Exercise Program for Individuals With Schizophrenia Spectrum Disorders." *The Journal of Nervous and Mental Disease* 204 (9): 651–57. https://doi.org/10.1097/NMD.0000000000000556.

Calne, D B. 1993. "Treatment of Parkinson's Disease." *The New England Journal of Medicine* 329 (14): 1021–27. https://doi.org/10.1056/NEJM199309303291408.

Casagrande, Sara Carvalho Barbosa, Rubens Gisbert Cury, Andrea Cristina de Lima-Pardini, Daniel Boari Coelho, Carolina de Oliveira Souza, Maria Gabriela Dos Santos Ghilardi, Laura Silveira-Moriyama, Luis Augusto Teixeira, Egberto Reis Barbosa, and Erich Talamoni Fonoff. 2017. "Dramatic Improvement of Tardive Dyskinesia Movements by Inline Skating." *Neurology* 89 (2): 211–13. https://doi.org/10.1212/WNL.0000000000004092.

Cohen, Ann D, Jennifer L Tillerson, Amanda D Smith, Timothy Schallert, and Michael J Zigmond. 2003. "Neuroprotective Effects of Prior Limb Use in 6-Hydroxydopamine-Treated Rats: Possible Role of GDNF." *Journal of Neurochemistry* 85 (2): 299–305.

d'Anglemont de Tassigny, Xavier, Alberto Pascual, and Jose Lopez-Barneo. 2015. "GDNF-Based Therapies, GDNF-Producing Interneurons, and Trophic Support of the Dopaminergic Nigrostriatal Pathway. Implications for Parkinson's Disease." *Frontiers in Neuroanatomy* 9: 10. https://doi.org/10.3389/fnana.2015.00010.

Dale, Russell C, Anna Melchers, Victor S C Fung, Padraic Grattan-Smith, Henry Houlden, and John Earl. 2010. "Familial Paroxysmal Exercise-Induced Dystonia: Atypical Presentation of Autosomal Dominant GTP-Cyclohydrolase 1 Deficiency." *Developmental Medicine and Child Neurology* 52 (6): 583–86. https://doi.org/10.1111/j.1469-8749.2010.03619.x.

Del-Bel, Elaine, Fernando E Padovan-Neto, Mariza Bortolanza, Vitor Tumas, Aderbal S Jr Aguiar, Rita Raisman-Vozari, and Rui D Prediger. 2015. "Nitric Oxide, a New Player in L-DOPA-Induced Dyskinesia?" *Frontiers in Bioscience (Elite Edition)* 7 (January): 168–92.

Demirkiran, M, and J Jankovic. 1995. "Paroxysmal Dyskinesias: Clinical Features and Classification." *Annals of Neurology* 38 (4): 571–79. https://doi.org/10.1002/ana.410380405.

Ellison, G, and R E See. 1989. "Rats Administered Chronic Neuroleptics Develop Oral Movements Which Are Similar in Form to Those in Humans with Tardive Dyskinesia." *Psychopharmacology* 98 (4): 564–66.

Fahn, S. 2000. "The Spectrum of Levodopa-Induced Dyskinesias." *Annals of Neurology* 47 (4 Suppl 1): S2-9; discussion S9-11.

Faurbye, A, P J Rasch, P B Petersen, G Brandborg, and H Pakkenberg. 1964. "Neurological Symptoms In Pharmacotherapy Of Psychoses." *Acta Psychiatrica Scandinavica* 40 (1): 10–27.

Fisher, Beth E, Giselle M Petzinger, Kerry Nixon, Elizabeth Hogg, Samuel Bremmer, Charles K Meshul, and Michael W Jakowec. 2004. "Exercise-Induced Behavioral Recovery and Neuroplasticity in the 1-Methyl-4-Phenyl-1,2,3,6-Tetrahydropyridine-Lesioned Mouse Basal Ganglia." *Journal of Neuroscience Research* 77 (3): 378–90. https://doi.org/10.1002/jnr.20162.

Fox, Susan H, Regina Katzenschlager, Shen-Yang Lim, Bernard Ravina, Klaus Seppi, Miguel Coelho, Werner Poewe, Olivier Rascol, Christopher G. Goetz, and Cristina Sampaio. 2011. "The Movement Disorder Society Evidence-Based Medicine Review Update: Treatments for the Motor Symptoms of Parkinson's Disease." *Movement Disorders* 26 (S3): S2–41. https://doi.org/10.1002/mds.23829.

Frazzitta, Giuseppe, Gabriella Bertotti, Micaela Morelli, Giulio Riboldazzi, Elisa Pelosin, Pietro Balbi, Natalia Boveri, et al. 2012. "Rehabilitation Improves Dyskinesias in Parkinsonian Patients: A Pilot Study Comparing Two Different Rehabilitative Treatments." *Neuro Rehabilitation* 30 (4): 295–301. https://doi.org/10.3233/NRE-2012-0758.

Frazzitta, Giuseppe, Micaela Morelli, Gabriella Bertotti, Guido Felicetti, Gianni Pezzoli, and Roberto Maestri. 2012. "Intensive Rehabilitation Treatment in Parkinsonian Patients with Dyskinesias: A Preliminary Study with 6-Month Followup." *Parkinson's Disease* 2012: 4–7. https://doi.org/10.1155/2012/910454.

Fredriksson, Anders, Ingels Maria Stigsdotter, Anders Hurtig, Beatrice Ewalds-Kvist, and Trevor Archer. 2011. "Running Wheel Activity Restores MPTP-Induced Functional Deficits." *Journal of Neural Transmission (Vienna, Austria : 1996)* 118 (3): 407–20. https://doi.org/10.1007/s00702-010-0474-8.

Friedman, Jennifer R, Aurelie Meneret, Dong-Hui Chen, Oriane Trouillard, Marie Vidailhet, Wendy H Raskind, and Emmanuel Roze. 2016. *ADCY5 Mutation Carriers Display Pleiotropic Paroxysmal Day and Nighttime Dyskinesias. Movement Disorders : Official Journal of the Movement Disorder Society.* Vol. 31. United States. https://doi.org/10.1002/mds.26494.

Ginovart, Nathalie, Alan A Wilson, Doug Hussey, Sylvain Houle, and Shitij Kapur. 2009. "D2-Receptor Upregulation Is Dependent upon Temporal Course of D2-Occupancy: A Longitudinal [11C]-Raclopride PET Study in Cats." *Neuropsychopharmacology : Official Publication of the American College of Neuropsychopharmacology* 34 (3): 662–71. https://doi.org/10.1038/npp.2008.116.

Goodenough, D J, R G Fariello, B L Annis, and R W Chun. 1978. "Familial and Acquired Paroxysmal Dyskinesias. A Proposed Classification with Delineation of Clinical Features." *Archives of Neurology* 35 (12): 827–31. https://doi.org/10.1001/archneur.1978.00500360051010.

Guerrini, R, P Bonanni, N Nardocci, L Parmeggiani, M Piccirilli, M De Fusco, P Aridon, A Ballabio, R Carrozzo, and G Casari. 1999. "Autosomal Recessive Rolandic Epilepsy with Paroxysmal Exercise-Induced Dystonia and Writer's Cramp: Delineation of the Syndrome and Gene Mapping to Chromosome 16p12-11.2." *Annals of Neurology* 45 (3): 344–52.

Haro, Josep Maria, and Luis Salvador-Carulla. 2006. "The SOHO (Schizophrenia Outpatient Health Outcome) Study: Implications for the Treatment of Schizophrenia." *CNS Drugs* 20 (4): 293–301. https://doi.org/10.2165/00023210-200620040-00003.

Hert, Marc DE, Christoph U Correll, Julio Bobes, Marcelo Cetkovich-Bakmas, Dan Cohen, Itsuo Asai, Johan Detraux, et al. 2011. "Physical Illness in Patients with Severe Mental Disorders. I. Prevalence, Impact of Medications and Disparities in Health Care." *World Psychiatry : Official Journal of the World Psychiatric Association (WPA)* 10 (1): 52–77.

Hjorth, Peter, Anette Juel, Mette Vinther Hansen, Nikolaj Juul Madsen, Anne Grethe Viuff, and Povl Munk-Jorgensen. 2017. "Reducing the

Risk of Cardiovascular Diseases in Non-Selected Outpatients With Schizophrenia: A 30-Month Program Conducted in a Real-Life Setting." *Archives of Psychiatric Nursing* 31 (6): 602–9. https://doi.org/10.1016/j.apnu.2017.08.005.

Horstink, M, E Tolosa, U Bonuccelli, G Deuschl, A Friedman, P Kanovsky, J P Larsen, et al. 2006. "Review of the Therapeutic Management of Parkinson's Disease. Report of a Joint Task Force of the European Federation of Neurological Societies (EFNS) and the Movement Disorder Society-European Section (MDS-ES). Part II: Late (Complicated) Parkinson's Dise." *European Journal of Neurology* 13 (11): 1186–1202. https://doi.org/10.1111/j.1468-1331.2006.01548.x.

Iravani, M M, S Costa, M J Jackson, B C Tel, C Cannizzaro, R K Pearce, and P Jenner. 2001. "GDNF Reverses Priming for Dyskinesia in MPTP-Treated, L-DOPA-Primed Common Marmosets." *The European Journal of Neuroscience* 13 (3): 597–608.

Jenner, Peter. 2008. "Molecular Mechanisms of L-DOPA-Induced Dyskinesia." *Nature Reviews. Neuroscience* 9 (9): 665–77. https://doi.org/10.1038/nrn2471.

Kaminer, Jaime, Pratibha Thakur, and Craig Evinger. 2015. "Effects of Subthalamic Deep Brain Stimulation on Blink Abnormalities of 6-OHDA Lesioned Rats." *Journal of Neurophysiology* 113 (9): 3038–46. https://doi.org/10.1152/jn.01072.2014.

Kieburtz, Karl. 2006. "Issues in Neuroprotection Clinical Trials in Parkinson's Disease." *Neurology* 66 (10 Suppl 4): S50-7.

Kim, Jungjin, Eric Macmaster, and Thomas L Schwartz. 2014. "Tardive Dyskinesia in Patients Treated with Atypical Antipsychotics: Case Series and Brief Review of Etiologic and Treatment Considerations." *Drugs in Context* 3: 212259. https://doi.org/10.7573/dic.212259.

Kirik, D, B Georgievska, C Rosenblad, and A Bjorklund. 2001. "Delayed Infusion of GDNF Promotes Recovery of Motor Function in the Partial Lesion Model of Parkinson's Disease." *The European Journal of Neuroscience* 13 (8): 1589–99.

Koning, Jeroen P F, Diederik E Tenback, Jim van Os, Andre Aleman, Rene S Kahn, and Peter N van Harten. 2010. "Dyskinesia and Parkinsonism in Antipsychotic-Naive Patients with Schizophrenia, First-Degree Relatives and Healthy Controls: A Meta-Analysis." *Schizophrenia Bulletin* 36 (4): 723–31. https://doi.org/10.1093/schbul/sbn146.

Kuo, Sheng-Han, and Joseph Jankovic. 2008. "Tardive Gait." *Clinical Neurology and Neurosurgery* 110 (2): 198–201. https://doi.org/10.1016/j.clineuro.2007.09.013.

Lance, J W. 1977. "Familial Paroxysmal Dystonic Choreoathetosis and Its Differentiation from Related Syndromes." *Annals of Neurology* 2 (4): 285–93. https://doi.org/10.1002/ana.410020405.

Lauterbach, E C, H Singh, G M Simpson, and R L Morrison. 1990. "Gait Disorders in Tardive Dyskinesia." *Acta Psychiatrica Scandinavica*. United States. https://doi.org/10.1111/j.1600-0447.1990.tb03065.x.

Lerner, Vladimir, and Chanoch Miodownik. 2011. "Motor Symptoms of Schizophrenia: Is Tardive Dyskinesia a Symptom or Side Effect? A Modern Treatment." *Current Psychiatry Reports* 13 (4): 295–304. https://doi.org/10.1007/s11920-011-0202-6.

Liu, Qing, Zhan Qi, Xin-Hua Wan, Jing-Yun Li, Lei Shi, Qiang Lu, Xiang-Qin Zhou, et al. 2012. "Mutations in PRRT2 Result in Paroxysmal Dyskinesias with Marked Variability in Clinical Expression." *Journal of Medical Genetics* 49 (2): 79–82. https://doi.org/10.1136/jmedgenet-2011-100653.

Mahmoudi, Souha, Daniel Levesque, and Pierre J Blanchet. 2014. "Upregulation of Dopamine D3, Not D2, Receptors Correlates with Tardive Dyskinesia in a Primate Model." *Movement Disorders : Official Journal of the Movement Disorder Society* 29 (9): 1125–33. https://doi.org/10.1002/mds.25909.

Mantri, Sneha, Michelle E Fullard, John E Duda, and James F Morley. 2018. "Physical Activity in Early Parkinson Disease." *Journal of Parkinson's Disease* 8 (1): 107–11. https://doi.org/10.3233/JPD-171218.

Meneret, A, and E Roze. 2016. "Paroxysmal Movement Disorders: An Update." *Revue Neurologique* 172 (8–9): 433–45. https://doi.org/10.1016/j.neurol.2016.07.005.

Merrill, Ray M, Joseph L Lyon, and Paul M Matiaco. 2013. "Tardive and Spontaneous Dyskinesia Incidence in the General Population." *BMC Psychiatry* 13 (May): 152. https://doi.org/10.1186/1471-244X-13-152.
Methapatara, Waritnan, and Manit Srisurapanont. 2011. "Pedometer Walking plus Motivational Interviewing Program for Thai Schizophrenic Patients with Obesity or Overweight: A 12-Week, Randomized, Controlled Trial." *Psychiatry and Clinical Neurosciences* 65 (4): 374–80. https://doi.org/10.1111/j.1440-1819.2011.02225.x.
Montero-Odasso, Manuel, Joe Verghese, Olivier Beauchet, and Jeffrey M Hausdorff. 2012. "Gait and Cognition: A Complementary Approach to Understanding Brain Function and the Risk of Falling." *Journal of the American Geriatrics Society* 60 (11): 2127–36. https://doi.org/10.1111/j.1532-5415.2012.04209.x.
Morris, J C, E H Rubin, E J Morris, and S A Mandel. 1987. "Senile Dementia of the Alzheimer's Type: An Important Risk Factor for Serious Falls." *Journal of Gerontology* 42 (4): 412–17. https://doi.org/10.1093/geronj/42.4.412.
Muller, Thomas, and Siegfried Muhlack. 2010. "Effect of Exercise on Reactivity and Motor Behaviour in Patients with Parkinson's Disease." *Journal of Neurology, Neurosurgery, and Psychiatry* 81 (7): 747–53. https://doi.org/10.1136/jnnp.2009.174987.
Munchau, A, E M Valente, G A Shahidi, L H Eunson, M G Hanna, N P Quinn, A H Schapira, N W Wood, and K P Bhatia. 2000. "A New Family with Paroxysmal Exercise Induced Dystonia and Migraine: A Clinical and Genetic Study." *Journal of Neurology, Neurosurgery, and Psychiatry* 68 (5): 609–14. https://doi.org/10.1136/jnnp.68.5.609.
Neville, B G, F M Besag, and C D Marsden. 1998. "Exercise Induced Steroid Dependent Dystonia, Ataxia, and Alternating Hemiplegia Associated with Epilepsy." *Journal of Neurology, Neurosurgery, and Psychiatry* 65 (2): 241–44. https://doi.org/10.1136/jnnp.65.2.241.
Parsons, B, D M Togasaki, S Kassir, and S Przedborski. 1995. "Neuroleptics Up-Regulate Adenosine A2a Receptors in Rat Striatum: Implications for the Mechanism and the Treatment of Tardive Dyskinesia." *Journal*

of Neurochemistry 65 (5): 2057–64. https://doi.org/10.1046/j.1471-4159.1995.65052057.x.

Roubergue, Anne, Emmanuel Roze, Sandrine Vuillaumier-Barrot, Marie-Josephine Fontenille, Aurelie Meneret, Marie Vidailhet, Bertrand Fontaine, et al. 2013. "The Multiple Faces of the ATP1A3-Related Dystonic Movement Disorder." *Movement Disorders : Official Journal of the Movement Disorder Society*. United States. https://doi.org/10.1002/mds.25396.

Schonecker, M. 1957. "[Paroxysmal dyskinesia as the effect of megaphen]." *Der Nervenarzt* 28 (12): 550–53.

Silvestri, S, M V Seeman, J C Negrete, S Houle, C M Shammi, G J Remington, S Kapur, et al. 2000. "Increased Dopamine D2 Receptor Binding after Long-Term Treatment with Antipsychotics in Humans: A Clinical PET Study." *Psychopharmacology* 152 (2): 174–80.

Simpson, G M, and R K Shrivastava. 1978. "Abnormal Gaits in Tardive Dyskinesia." *The American Journal of Psychiatry*. United States. https://doi.org/10.1176/ajp.135.7.865a.

Speck, Ana E, Marissa G Schamne, Aderbal Jr S Aguiar, Rodrigo A Cunha, and Rui D Prediger. 2018. "Treadmill Exercise Attenuates L-DOPA-Induced Dyskinesia and Increases Striatal Levels of Glial Cell-Derived Neurotrophic Factor (GDNF) in Hemiparkinsonian Mice." *Molecular Neurobiology*, August. https://doi.org/10.1007/s12035-018-1278-3.

Stacy, M, F Cardoso, and J Jankovic. 1993. "Tardive Stereotypy and Other Movement Disorders in Tardive Dyskinesias." *Neurology* 43 (5): 937–41. https://doi.org/10.1212/wnl.43.5.937.

Standaert, David G, Ramon L Rodriguez, John T Slevin, Michael Lobatz, Susan Eaton, Krai Chatamra, Maurizio F Facheris, et al. 2017. "Effect of Levodopa-Carbidopa Intestinal Gel on Non-Motor Symptoms in Patients with Advanced Parkinson's Disease." *Movement Disorders Clinical Practice* 4 (6): 829–37. https://doi.org/10.1002/mdc3.12526.

Strassnig, Martin, Jaspreet S Brar, and Rohan Ganguli. 2011. "Low Cardiorespiratory Fitness and Physical Functional Capacity in Obese Patients with Schizophrenia." *Schizophrenia Research* 126 (1–3): 103–9. https://doi.org/10.1016/j.schres.2010.10.025.

Strassnig, Martin, Amie Rosenfeld, and Philip D Harvey. 2018. "Tardive Dyskinesia: Motor System Impairments, Cognition and Everyday Functioning." *CNS Spectrums* 23 (6): 370–77. https://doi.org/10.1017/S1092852917000542.

Stubbs, Brendon, Joseph Firth, Alexandra Berry, Felipe B Schuch, Simon Rosenbaum, Fiona Gaughran, Nicola Veronesse, et al. 2016. "How Much Physical Activity Do People with Schizophrenia Engage in? A Systematic Review, Comparative Meta-Analysis and Meta-Regression." *Schizophrenia Research* 176 (2–3): 431–40. https://doi.org/10.1016/j.schres.2016.05.017.

Stubbs, Brendon, Ai Koyanagi, Felipe Schuch, Joseph Firth, Simon Rosenbaum, Fiona Gaughran, James Mugisha, and Davy Vancampfort. 2017. "Physical Activity Levels and Psychosis: A Mediation Analysis of Factors Influencing Physical Activity Target Achievement Among 204 186 People Across 46 Low- and Middle-Income Countries." *Schizophrenia Bulletin* 43 (3): 536–45. https://doi.org/10.1093/schbul/sbw111.

Tarsy, Daniel, and Ross J Baldessarini. 2006. "Epidemiology of Tardive Dyskinesia: Is Risk Declining with Modern Antipsychotics?" *Movement Disorders : Official Journal of the Movement Disorder Society* 21 (5): 589–98. https://doi.org/10.1002/mds.20823.

Tarsy, Daniel, Codrin Lungu, and Ross J Baldessarini. 2011. "Epidemiology of Tardive Dyskinesia before and during the Era of Modern Antipsychotic Drugs." *Handbook of Clinical Neurology* 100: 601–16. https://doi.org/10.1016/B978-0-444-52014-2.00043-4.

Tinetti, M E, M Speechley, and S F Ginter. 1988. "Risk Factors for Falls among Elderly Persons Living in the Community." *The New England Journal of Medicine* 319 (26): 1701–7. https://doi.org/10.1056/NEJM198812293192604.

Toy, William A, Giselle M Petzinger, Brian J Leyshon, Garnik K Akopian, P John, Matilde V Hoffman, Marta G Vu, and Michael W Jakowec. 2014. "*Treadmill Exercise Reverses Dendritic Spine Loss in Direct and Indirect Striatal Medium Spiny Neurons in the 1-Methyl-4- Phenyl-1,2,3,6-Tetrahydropyridine (MPTP) Mouse Model of Parkinson's*

Disease - *ARTIGO NOVO*," 201–9. https://doi.org/10.1016/j.nbd. 2013.11.017.Treadmill.

Verghese, Joe, Jeannette Mahoney, Anne F Ambrose, Cuiling Wang, and Roee Holtzer. 2010. "Effect of Cognitive Remediation on Gait in Sedentary Seniors." *The Journals of Gerontology. Series A, Biological Sciences and Medical Sciences* 65 (12): 1338–43. https://doi.org/10.1093/gerona/glq127.

Vuckovic, Marta G, Quanzheng Li, Beth Fisher, Angelo Nacca, Richard M Leahy, John P Walsh, Jogesh Mukherjee, Celia Williams, Michael W Jakowec, and Giselle M Petzinger. 2010. "Exercise Elevates Dopamine D2 Receptor in a Mouse Model of Parkinson's Disease: In Vivo Imaging with [(1)(8)F]Fallypride." *Movement Disorders : Official Journal of the Movement Disorder Society* 25 (16): 2777–84. https://doi.org/10.1002/mds.23407.

Waddington, J L. 1989. "Schizophrenia, Affective Psychoses, and Other Disorders Treated with Neuroleptic Drugs: The Enigma of Tardive Dyskinesia, Its Neurobiological Determinants, and the Conflict of Paradigms." *International Review of Neurobiology* 31: 297–353.

———. 1990. "Spontaneous Orofacial Movements Induced in Rodents by Very Long-Term Neuroleptic Drug Administration: Phenomenology, Pathophysiology and Putative Relationship to Tardive Dyskinesia." *Psychopharmacology* 101 (4): 431–47.

Wang, Libo, Jia Li, and Jiajun Chen. 2018. "Levodopa-Carbidopa Intestinal Gel in Parkinson's Disease: A Systematic Review and Meta-Analysis." *Frontiers in Neurology* 9: 620. https://doi.org/10.3389/fneur.2018.00620.

Weber, Y G, C Kamm, A Suls, J Kempfle, K Kotschet, R Schule, T V Wuttke, et al. 2011. "Paroxysmal Choreoathetosis/Spasticity (DYT9) Is Caused by a GLUT1 Defect." *Neurology* 77 (10): 959–64. https://doi.org/10.1212/WNL.0b013e31822e0479.

Wilcox, P G, A Bassett, B Jones, and J A Fleetham. 1994. "Respiratory Dysrhythmias in Patients with Tardive Dyskinesia." *Chest* 105 (1): 203–7. https://doi.org/10.1378/chest.105.1.203.

Wolf, M A, R Yassa, and P M Llorca. 1993. "[Neuroleptic-induced movement disorders: historical perspectives]." *L'Encephale* 19 (6): 657–61.

Wu, Meng Hsiu, Chin Pang Lee, Shih Chieh Hsu, Chia Ming Chang, and Ching Yen Chen. 2015. "Effectiveness of High-Intensity Interval Training on the Mental and Physical Health of People with Chronic Schizophrenia." *Neuropsychiatric Disease and Treatment* 11: 1255–63. https://doi.org/10.2147/NDT.S81482.

Yassa, R. 1989. "Functional Impairment in Tardive Dyskinesia: Medical and Psychosocial Dimensions." *Acta Psychiatrica Scandinavica* 80 (1): 64–67. https://doi.org/10.1111/j.1600-0447.1989.tb01301.x.

Yassa, R, and B D Jones. 1985. "Complications of Tardive Dyskinesia: A Review." *Psychosomatics* 26 (4): 305-307,310,312-313. https://doi.org/10.1016/S0033-3182(85)72863-0.

Zorzi, G, B Castellotti, F Zibordi, C Gellera, and N Nardocci. 2008. "Paroxysmal Movement Disorders in GLUT1 Deficiency Syndrome." *Neurology* 71 (2): 146–48. https://doi.org/10.1212/01.wnl.0000316804.10020.ba.

Zukerman, E, L C Vilanova, and J Serafico. 1983. "[Familial paroxysmal choreoathetosis. Report of 2 cases in one family]." *Arquivos de neuro-psiquiatria* 41 (4): 373–76.

BIBLIOGRAPHY

A guide to the extrapyramidal side-effects of antipsychotic drugs
LCCN	2013039676
Type of material	Book
Personal name	Owens, D. G. Cunningham (David Griffith Cunningham), 1949- author.
Main title	A guide to the extrapyramidal side-effects of antipsychotic drugs / D. G. Cunningham-Owens, Professor of Clinical Psychiatry, University of Edinburgh, Division of Psychiatry, Royal Edinburgh Hospital, Edinburgh, UK.
Edition	Second edition.
Published/Produced	Cambridge; New York: Cambridge University Press, [2014] ©2014
Description	viii, 377 pages: illustrations; 26 cm
ISBN	9781107022867 (hardback) 110702286X (hardback)
LC classification	RM333.5 .O94 2014
Summary	"It is often implied that antipsychotic-induced extrapyramidal side-effects are irrelevant to

modern psychiatric therapeutics, rendered historic by newer, better treatments. This myth arises from limited awareness of the depth and breadth of neurological disruption antipsychotics can mediate. This volume discusses the extensive clinical boundaries of acute dystonias, drug-induced parkinsonism, akathisia and tardive dyskinesia, providing demographic and epidemiological context while illustrating how prescribing choices impact powerfully on their development. This new edition has been thoroughly updated and rewritten to include recent data, expanded references and a new chapter on the concept of 'atypical' antipsychotics. Written in a light, engaging style, liberally illustrated with clinical examples, it also invites readers to consider ongoing controversies - subjective drug effects, the relationship between 'akathisia' and restless legs, the status of the concept of 'atypicality', and so on. Informative reading for trainees as well as established practitioners in the fields of psychiatry, neurology, primary care and geriatrics"--Provided by publisher.

Contents   Preface; Part 1. Setting the Scene: 1. The origins of psychopharma; 2. Some preliminaries; Part 2. The Syndromes: 3. Acute dystonias; 4. Parkinsonism; 5. Akathisia; 6. Tardive dyskinesia; Part 3. Particular Issues: 7. Tardive and chronic dystonia; 8. Special populations; Part 4. Assessment: 9. The clinical examination; 10. An overview of some standardised recording instruments; Part 5. Matters Arising: 11. Involuntary movements and schizophrenia: a

Subjects	limitation to the concept of tardive dyskinesia?; 12. And finally ... the salutary tale of 'atypicality'; References; Index. Basal Ganglia Diseases--chemically induced. Antipsychotic Agents--adverse effects. Extrapyramidal Tracts--drug effects. Neurotoxicity Syndromes.
Notes	Includes bibliographical references (pages 320-370) and index.

Brain stimulation

LCCN	2013481862
Type of material	Book
Uniform title	Brain stimulation (Lozano)
Main title	Brain stimulation / volume editors, Andres M. Lozano, Mark Hallett.
Published/Produced	Edinburgh; London; New York; Oxford; Philadelphia; St. Louis; Sydney; Toronto: Elsevier, 2013.
Description	xx, 763 pages: illustrations (chiefly color); 27 cm.
Links	Publisher description http://www.loc.gov/catdir/enhancements/fy1606/2013481862-d.html
ISBN	9780444534972 0444534970
LC classification	RC350.B72 B735 2013
Related names	Lozano, A. M. (Andres M.), 1959- editor. Hallett, Mark, 1943- editor.
Summary	"The field of brain stimulation is expanding rapidly, with techniques such as DBS, TMS, and tDCS moving from the research community into clinical diagnosis and treatment. Clinical applications include treating disorders such as Parkinson's disease, dystonia, and even depression" -- Publisher's description.

Contents Sect. 1. Deep brain stimulation -- Principles of electrical simulations of neural tissue -- Deep brain stimulation in animal models -- Deep brain stimulation surgical techniques -- Deep brain stimulation: how does it work? -- Computational modeling of deep brain stimulation -- Therapeutic stimulation versus ablation -- Magnetic resonance imaging safety of deep brain stimulator devices -- Brain stimulation and functional imaging with fMRI and PET -- Deep brain stimulation for Parkinson's disease: patient selection -- Clinical outcome of deep brain stimulation for Parkinson's disease -- Postoperative management of deep brain stimulation in Parkinson's disease -- Psychiatric considerations in deep brain stimulation for Parkinson's disease -- Deep brain stimulation for essential tremor -- Deep brain stimulation for dystonia -- Role of deep brain stimulation in the treatment of secondary dystonia-dyskinesia syndromes -- Deep brain stimulation for other tremor, myoclonus, and chorea -- Deep brain stimulation for epilepsy -- Deep brain stimulation for major depression -- Deep brain stimulation in obsessive-compulsive disorder: neurocircuitry and clinical experience -- Deep brain stimulation for Tourette syndrome -- Deep brain stimulation in addiction due to psychoactive substance use -- Evaluating the potential of deep brain stimulation for treatment-resistant anorexia nervosa -- Deep brain stimulation for pain -- Central thalamic deep brain stimulation for support of forebrain arousal regulation in the minimally conscious state -- Deep brain stimulation for cognitive disorders --

Ethics guidance for neurological and psychiatric deep brain stimulation -- Sect. 2. Superficial brain stimulation -- Transcranial electric and magnetic stimulation: technique and paradigms -- Epidural and subdural stimulation -- Physics of effects of transcranial brain stimulation -- Biological effects of non-invasive brain stimulation -- Central motor conduction time -- Pharmaco-transcranial magnetic stimulation studies of motor excitability -- Treating the depressions with superficial brain stimulation methods -- Other therapeutic psychiatric uses of superficial brain stimulation -- Pain -- Tinnitus: therapeutic use of superficial brain stimulation -- Parkinson's disease -- Dystonia -- Epilepsy -- Noninvasive brain stimulation in neurorehabilitation -- Plasticity -- Parkinson's disease -- Transcranial magnetic stimulation in dystonia -- Noninvasive brain stimulation in Huntington's disease -- Utility of transcranial magnetic stimulation in delineating amyotrophic lateral sclerosis pathophysiology -- Superficial brain stimulation in multiple sclerosis -- Brain stimulation in migraine -- Dementia -- Addiction -- Tourette syndrome -- Cerebellum -- Transcranial magnetic stimulation and vision -- Transcranial magnetic stimulation techniques to study the somatosensory system: research applications -- Language -- Learning and memory -- Transcranial stimulation and cognition.

Subjects Brain stimulation.
Brain stimulation--Therapeutic use.
Deep Brain Stimulation.
Mental Disorders--therapy.
Nervous System Diseases--therapy.

Notes	Transcranial Magnetic Stimulation. Includes bibliographical references and index.
Additional formats	Online version: Brain stimulation. Amsterdam: Elsevier, 2013 9780444534989 (OCoLC)861797691
Series	Handbook of clinical neurology; volume 116, 3rd series

Case studies: Stahl's essential psychopharmacology

LCCN	2011006215
Type of material	Book
Personal name	Stahl, Stephen M., 1951-
Main title	Case studies: Stahl's essential psychopharmacology / Stephen M. Stahl.
Published/Created	Cambridge, UK; New York: Cambridge University Press, 2011.
Description	xxiii, 485 p.: ill. (some col.); 23 cm.
ISBN	9780521182089 (pbk.)
LC classification	RC483 .S66 2011
Portion of title	Stahl's essential psychopharmacology
Summary	"Designed with the distinctive, user-friendly presentation Dr Stahl's audience know and love, this new stream of Stahl books capitalize on Dr Stahl's greatest strength - the ability to address complex issues in an understandable way and with direct relevance to the everyday experience of clinicians. The book describes a wide-ranging and representative selection of clinical scenarios, making use of icons, questions/answers and tips. It follows these cases through the complete clinical encounter, from start to resolution, acknowledging all the complications, issues, decisions, twists and turns along the way. The book is about living through the treatments that

work, the treatments that fail, and the mistakes made along the journey. This is psychiatry in real life - these are the patients from your waiting room - this book will reassure, inform and guide better clinical decision making"--Provided by publisher.

Contents

1. The man whose antidepressants stopped working; 2. The son who would not take a shower; 3. The man who kept hitting his wife over the head with a frying pan; 4. The son who could not go to bed; 5. The sleepy woman with anxiety; 6. The woman who felt numb; 7. The case of physician do not heal thyself; 8. The son whose parents were desperate to have him avoid Kraepelin; 9. The soldier who thinks he is a 'slacker' broken beyond all repair after 3 deployments to Iraq; 10. The young man everybody was afraid to treat; 11. The young woman whose doctors could not decide whether she has schizophrenia, bipolar disorder or both; 12. The scary man with only partial symptom control on clozapine; 13. The 8 year old girl who was naughty; 14. The scatter-brained mother whose daughter has ADHD, like mother, like daughter; 15. The doctor who couldn't keep up with his patients; 16. The computer analyst who thought the government would choke him to death; 17. The severely depressed man with a life insurance policy soon to lose its suicide exemption; 18. The anxious woman who was more afraid of her anxiety medications than of anything else; 19. The psychotic woman with delusions that no medication could fix; 20. The breast cancer survivor who couldn't remember how to cook; 21. The woman who has always

	been out of control; 22. The young man with depression and alcohol abuse -- like father, like son, like grandfather, like father, like great grandfather, like grandfather; 23. The woman with psychotic depression responsive to her own TMS machine; 24. The boy getting kicked out of his classroom; 25. The young man whose dyskinesia was prompt and not tardive; 26. The patient whose daughter wouldn't give up; 27. The psychotic arsonist who burned his house and tried to burn himself; 28. The woman with depression whose Parkinson's Disease vanished; 29. The depressed man who thought he was out of options; 30. The woman who was either manic or fat; 31. The girl who couldn't find a doctor; 32. The man who wondered if once a bipolar always a bipolar?; 33. Suck it up, soldier, and quit whining; 34. The young man who is failing to launch; 35. The young cancer survivor with panic; 36. The man whose antipsychotic almost killed him; 37. The painful man who soaked up his opiates like a sponge; 38. The woman with an ever fluctuating mood; 39. The psychotic sex offender with grandiosity and mania; 40. The elderly man with schizophrenia and Alzheimer's Disease; Index.
Subjects	Mental illness--Chemotherapy--Case studies.
Mental illness--Chemotherapy--Examinations, questions, etc.
Psychopharmacology--Case studies.
Psychopharmacology--Examinations, questions, etc.
Mental Disorders--drug therapy--Case Reports.
Mental Disorders--drug therapy--Examination Questions.

	Psychopharmacology--methods--Case Reports.
	Psychopharmacology--methods--Examination Questions.
Notes	Includes bibliographical references and indexes.

Case studies in movement disorders: common and uncommon presentations

LCCN	2017000344
Type of material	Book
Main title	Case studies in movement disorders: common and uncommon presentations / edited by Roberto Erro, Center for Neurodegenerative Diseases (CEMAND), Department of Medicine and Surgery, Neuroscience Section, University of Salerno, Italy, Sobell Department of Movement Disorders and Motor Neuroscience, Institute of Neurology, UCL, London, UK, Maria Stamelou, University of Athens Medical School, 2nd Department of Neurology, Hospital Attikon, Athens, Greece, Movement Disorders Department, HYGEIA Hospital, Athens, Greece, Department of Neurology, Philipps University, Marburg, Germany, Kailash P. Bhatia, Sobell Department of Movement Disorders and Motor Neuroscience, Institute of Neurology, UCL, London, UK.
Published/Produced	Cambridge, United Kingdom; New York, NY: Cambridge University Press, 2017.
Description	xx, 154 pages: illustrations (some color); 25 cm.
ISBN	9781107472426 (paperback)
	1107472423
LC classification	RC376.5 .C375 2017
Related names	Bhatia, Kailash, editor.
	Erro, Roberto, editor.

Summary	Stamelou, Maria, editor.
"Drawing on the expertise of an international team of authors, Case Studies in Movement Disorders is a compilation of illustrative cases, demonstrating a step-by-step approach to diagnosing and managing these complex conditions. An extensive collection of over sixty videos shows both common and uncommon presentations of a wide-range of movement disorders, and the accompanying text guides readers systematically through the clinical history, examination and investigation findings, diagnosis, and finally discusses the clinical issues raised. Both surgical and pharmacological management options are presented, helping readers understand some of the controversies involved in treatment. The cases are drawn from all of the major groups of movement disorders: ataxia, chorea, dystonia, myoclonus, parkinsonism, tics, and tremor. This will be invaluable for both neurologists in training and more experienced professionals seeking to develop their diagnostic skills, especially when faced with uncommon conditions or uncommon manifestations of common disorders"-- Provided by publisher.
Contents	List of contributors; List of abbreviations; Section 1. Parkinsonism: 1. Parkinson disease; 2. Nonmotor Parkinson disease; 3. Isolated lower limb dystonia at onset of Parkin disease; 4. Parkinson's disease associated with SCNA mutations; 5. Steele-Richardson-Olszewski syndrome; 6. PSP-Parkinsonism; 7. Corticobasal degeneration; 8. MSA - Parkinsonian variant; 9.

Prominent freezing of gait and speech disturbances due to Fahr disease; 10. A (familial) PSP-look alike; 11. Parkinsonian syndrome and sunflower cataracts: Wilson's disease; 12. Classic PD-like rest tremor in FTDP-17 due to a MAPT mutation; 13. Progressive parkinsonism with falls and supranuclear gaze palsy; 14. Very early onset parkinsonism; 15. Parkinsonism due to CSF1R mutation; Section 2. Dystonia: 16. Early-onset generalized dystonia: DYT1; 17. Early-onset jerky dystonia: an uncommon phenotype of DYT1; 18. Early-onset generalized dystonia with cranio-cervical involvement: DYT6; 19. Autosomal recessive isolated generalized dystonia: DYT2; 20. Dopa-responsive dystonia; 21. A complicated dopa-responsive dystonia: tyrosine hydroxylase deficiency; 22. Early onset generalized dystonia and macrocephaly: Glutaric Aciduria type 1; 23. PKAN misdiagnosed as "Progressive Delayed-Onset Postanoxic Dystonia"; 24. Oromandibular dystonia and freezing of gait: a novel presentation of neuroferritinopathy; 25. Generalized dystonia with oromandibular involvement and self-mutilations: Lesch-Nyhan sydnrome; 26. Dystonia complicated by pyramidal signs, parkinsonism and cognitive impairment: HSP11; 27. H-ABC syndrome; 28. Dystonic opisthotonus; 29. Delayed-onset dystonia after lightning strike; Section 3. Tics: 30. Gilles de la Tourette syndrome; 31. Secondary tic disorders: Huntington disease; 32. Multiple hyperkinesias: tics and paroxysmal kinesigenic dyskinesia; 33. Functional tic disorders; Section 4. Chorea: 34.

Huntington disease; 35. Generalized chorea with oromandibular involvement and tongue biting; 36. A Huntington disease look-alike: SCA17; 37. A newly recognized HD-phenocopy associated with C9orf72 expansion; 38. Persistent chorea due to anticholinergics in DYT6; 39. Dyskinesia without levodopa: long-term follow-up of mesencephalic transplant in PD; 40. Benign Hereditary Chorea; 41. Another cause of Benign Hereditary Chorea; Section 5. Tremor: 42. Essential Tremor; 43. Rest Tremor and Scans without evidence of dopaminergic deficit (SWEDD); 44. Neuropathic Tremor; 45. A treatable disorder misdiagnosed as ET; 46. Thalamic tremor; 47. Shaking on standing: orthostatic tremor; 48. Palatal tremor; 49. Dystonic tremor and progressive ataxia; 50. Bilateral Holmes tremor in Multiple Sclerosis; 51. Primary writing tremor; Section 6. Myoclonus: 52. A case of "essential" myoclonus; 53. Ramsey Hunt syndrome and Unverricht-Lundborg disease; 54. North Sea Myoclonus due to GOSR2 mutations; 55. Ramsay Hunt syndrome and coeliac disease; 56. Asymmetric myoclonus and apraxia: Corticobasal syndromep; 57. Rapidly progressive cognitive regression and myoclonus; 58. Familial cortical "tremor"; 59. Prominent myoclonus and parkinsonism; 60. Axial myoclonus of uncertain origin; Section 7. Ataxia: 61. Slowly progressive unsteadiness and double vision; 62. Cerebellar ataxia with urinary incontinence: MSA-C; 63. Progressive ataxia, tremor, autonomic dysfunction and cognitive impairment; 64. Sensory ataxic neuropathy with

	dysarthria and ophthalmoparesis (SANDO) syndrome; 65. Ataxia Telangiectasia without ataxia; 66. Anti-Yo related ataxia misdiagnosed as Multiple System Atrophy; 67. Late onset spinocerebellar ataxia; 68. Ataxia with splenomegaly: Niemann-Pick disease type C.
Subjects	Movement disorders.
	Movement disorders--Case studies.
	Medical / Neurology.
Notes	Includes bibliographical references and index.
Series	Cambridge medicine

Clinical canine and feline respiratory medicine

LCCN	2009049308
Type of material	Book
Personal name	Johnson, Lynelle R.
Main title	Clinical canine and feline respiratory medicine / Lynelle R. Johnson.
Published/Created	Ames, Iowa: Wiley-Blackwell, c2010.
Description	xi, 202 p.: col. ill.; 25 cm.
ISBN	9780813816715 (pbk.: alk. paper)
LC classification	SF992.R47 J64 2010
Summary	"Clinical Canine and Feline Respiratory Disease provides reliable information on respiratory diagnosis and disease in a user-friendly format. With an emphasis on the features of the history and physical examination that aid in efficient treatment planning, the book is an accessible, readable resource to treating patients with diseases of the respiratory tract. Offering more comprehensive coverage of respiratory disorders than is available in general texts, Clinical Canine and Feline Respiratory Disease is specifically designed as a study aid and practice guide for the

Contents

non-specialist seeing respiratory cases. Beginning with introductory chapters on the localization of disease, diagnostics, and therapeutics, the heart of the book focuses on the full range of respiratory diseases. Coverage includes nasal disorders, diseases of airways, parenchymal diseases, pleural and mediastinal diseases, and vascular disorders. Clinical Canine and Feline Respiratory Disease is a useful tool to students and practitioners in studying, diagnosing, and treating respiratory disease"--Provided by publisher.
1. Localization of disease: use history and physical examination to characterize upper vs. lower, airway vs. parenchymal vs. pleural, heart vs. lung,.2. Respiratory diagnostics:.General: lab work and serology, pulse oximetry, arterial blood gas analysis, ECG?.Imaging: radiography, fluoroscopy, US and CT, transoral and transtracheal wash, respiratory endoscopy, thoracocentesis, FNA and lung biopsy, scintigraphy.Sample analysis: nasal/airway/fluid cytology and culture.3. Respiratory therapeutics:.Specific drugs: antibiotics, antifungals, glucocorticoids, bronchodilators, mucolytics.Routes of therapy: parenteral vs. enteral, nebulization, metered dose inhalers.Adjunct therapy: coupage, nutritional management, oxygen administration, indications for ventilatory support, chest tube placement..Disease sections below to include brief history and physical exam features specific for each disorder, relevant pathophysiology, specific diagnostic findings, treatment, prognosis..4. Nasal disorders.Structural: stenotic

	nares and brachycephalic syndrome, nasal foreign body, tooth root abscess, nasopharyngeal stenosis.Infectious: Cryptococcosis, aspergillosis.Inflammatory: nasopharyngeal polyps, CRS, LPR.Neoplastic.5. Diseases of airways.Structural: laryngeal paralysis, tracheal collapse, bronchiectasis.Infectious: canine upper respiratory disease complex (expand to include Bordetella and Mycoplasma bronchitis), parasitic bronchitis.Inflammatory: chronic bronchitis, feline asthma/bronchitis.Neoplastic.6. Parenchymal disease.Structural: ciliary dyskinesia, lung lobe torsion.Infectious: pneumonia (bacterial, fungal, viral, rickettsial, protozoal).Inflammatory: eosinophilic bronchopneumopathy, aspiration pneumonia, pulmonary fibrosis.Neoplastic.7. Pleural and mediastinal disease.Structural: pneumothorax, diaphragmatic hernia.Infectious: pyothorax, FIP.Neoplastic.Miscellaneous: hemothorax, chylothorax.8. Vascular disorders: pulmonary thromboembolism, heartworm disease, pulmonary hypertension.
Subjects	Respiratory organs--Diseases. Dogs--Diseases. Cats--Diseases. Dog Diseases--therapy. Respiratory Tract Diseases--veterinary. Cat Diseases--therapy. Clinical Medicine--methods.
Notes	Includes bibliographical references and index.

Deep brain stimulation: a case-based approach

LCCN	2019059949
Type of material	Book
Main title	Deep brain stimulation: a case-based approach / Shilpa Chitnis.
Published/Produced	New York, NY: Oxford University Press, [2020]
Description	1 online resource
ISBN	9780190647230 (other)
	9780190647223 (epub)
	(hardback)
LC classification	RC350.B72
Related names	Chitnis, Shilpa, editor.
	Khemani, Pravin, editor.
	Okun, Michael S., editor.
Summary	"Tremor is an involuntary movement characterized by a rhythmic oscillation about a fixed point or trajectory. It can be classified based on its clinical features or underlying cause. Tremor was the first approved indication for DBS in the U.S. We now have almost three decades of experience of tremor treatment with DBS. Essential tremor (ET) is the most frequent movement disorder occurring at a frequency of about 5 times that of PD. ET commonly has an autosomal dominant transmission pattern with incomplete penetrance, therefore sporadic cases are not at all uncommon. In ET, most patients suffer from tremor of the hands and arms; approximately 40% suffer from head and 20% from voice tremor. The majority of candidates for functional neurosurgery belong to the ET subgroup which is commonly characterized by severe action or postural tremor that impairs function and quality of life to the extent that the

risks, costs and inconvenience of DBS treatment are justified. Unilateral procedures (targeting the thalamus contralateral to the dominant and/or most affected hand) are commonly performed, though bilateral procedures should be considered when limb tremor is severe bilaterally, or when head, voice, or trunk tremors cause significant disability"-- Provided by publisher.

Contents

Introduction to creative programming techniques / Meagen Salinas -- Candidate selection for essential tremor / Laura Surillo Dahdah -- DBS programming for essential tremor / Brent Bluett -- Utilizing DBS to improve orthostatic tremor / Anhar Hassan -- Bilateral VIM-Thalamic DBS for medication-refractory orthostatic tremor / Mitra Afshari & Jill Ostrem -- Rebound tremor following a sub-optimally placed VIM DBS / Parul Jindal & Joohi Jimenez-Shahed -- Symptomatic cystic lesion following DBS surgery / Vibhash Sharma & Shilpa Chitnis -- Candidate selection for DBS for Parkinson's disease / Laura Surillo Dahdah -- DBS Programming for Parkinson's disease / Raja Mehanna -- Target selection for Parkinson's disease with medication refractory unilateral resting tremor / Fuyuko Sasaki & Genko Oyama -- Genetic mutations and DBS / Jared Hinkle & Zoltan Mari -- Issues to consider when mild cognitive impairment is revealed in pre-operative screening / Sushma Kola & Anhar Hassan -- Use of the STN and GPi deep brain stimulation targets in the same Parkinson's patient: patient specific targeting / Shabbir Hussain I. Merchant & Nora Vanegas-Arroyave -- Medication-refractory

Parkinsonian tremor requiring dual lead implantation for tremor control / Anhar Hassan -- Use of constant current mode to allow both monopolar and bipolar interleaving at a single contact / Meredith Spindler & Lana Chahine -- STN-DBS may improve pain in the setting of Parkinson's disease / Anjali Gera, Gian Pal -- DBS responsive camptocormia in Parkinson's disease / Elena Call & Helen Bronte-Stewart -- Deactivation of one STN-DBS device to address brittle ipsilateral dyskinesia in a patient with tremor-dominant Parkinson's disease / Julia Kroth & Sergiu Groppa -- Management of stimulation-induced dyskinesia in Parkinson disease with interleaving programming settings / Vibhash Sharma & Rajesh Pahwa -- Management of brittle dyskinesia and DDS in subthalamic deep brain stimulation / Junaid Siddiqui & Jawad Bajwa -- Freezing of Gait after Bilateral GPi-DBS in generalized dystonia / Mariana Moskovich -- GPi stimulation-induced gait disturbance and management by re-programming / Dhanya Vijayakumar & Joohi Jimenez-Shahed -- Rescue Vim DBS to address refractory tremor following STN DBS with brittle stimulation-induced dyskinesia / Mitra Afshari & Jill Ostrem -- Postural instability and gait disorder after STN-DBS: Evaluating disease progression, stimulation settings and medication / Javier R. Pérez-Sánchez & Monica M. Kurtis -- Non-surgical management of an exposed DBS lead / Ethan G. Brown & Jill Ostrem -- Steroid-responsive edema interfering with DBS programming / Pravin Khemani & Shilpa Chitnis -- The positive lesion effects of intracranial hemorrhage on DBS surgery outcome / Jacqueline Meystedt & David Charles -- Fibrous scarring and DBS lead implantation / Vinata Vedam Mai & Michael Okun -- Cerebral venous infarction after deep brain stimulation surgery / Andi Nugraha Sendjaja & Takashi Morishita -- Open circuits and loss of DBS benefit in the setting of Parkinson's disease / Arjun Tarakad & Joohi Jimenez-Shahed -- Acute neuropsychiatric symptoms and impulse control disorders after subthalamic nucleus deep brain stimulation / Adolfo Ramirez-Zamora & Michael Okun -- Improved outcome on interleaved deep brain stimulation settings / Svjetlana Miocinovic & Shilpa Chitnis -- Deep brain stimulation targeting the ventral intermediate nucleus of the thalamus for Parkinsonian tremor and later adding the the globus pallidus internus for Parkinson's disease features / Teri Thompsen -- Expected improvement in sleep quality and unexpected improvement in severe nightmares after DBS in Parkinson's disease / Laurice Yang -- Candidate selection for DBS for dystonia / Laura Surillo Dah Dah -- DBS programming for dystonia / Mitesh Lotia -- Choosing a target for DBS in dystonia associated tremor: GPi, VIM, STN, Zi or a combination of targets / Mustafa Siddiqui & Stephen B. Tatter -- Stimulation induced dyskinesia, interleaving settings and management of STN DBS in DYT-1 dystonia / Kyle T. Mitchell & Jill Ostrem -- Deep brain stimulation targeting the globus pallidus internus for dystonic tremor in the setting of generalized dystonia / Teri Thompsen -- Huntington's disease: DBS in adult

	Huntington's disease for treatment of axial dystonia / Jessica A. Carl and Leo Verhagen Metman -- Aggressiveness: DBS for medically refractory aggressive and injurious behavior / Oscar Bernal-Pacheco -- Bilateral globus pallidus DBS for dystonia and dystonic tremor in spinocerebellar ataxia 17 / Aparna Shukla and Pam Zeilman -- Deep Brain Stimulation for disabling "outflow" tremors: troubleshooting strategies for tremor habituation / Corneliu Luca -- Tardive dystonia and dyskinesia responsive to deep brain stimulation / Irene Malaty.
Subjects	Brain stimulation--Therapeutic use--Case studies. Extrapyramidal disorders--Treatment--Case studies. Tremor--Treatment--Case studies. Nervous system--Surgery--Case studies.
Notes	Includes bibliographical references and index.
Additional formats	Print version: Deep brain stimulation New York, NY: Oxford University Press, [2020] 9780190647209 (DLC) 2019059948

Deep brain stimulation: a case-based approach

LCCN	2019059948
Type of material	Book
Main title	Deep brain stimulation: a case-based approach / Shilpa Chitnis, Pravin Khemani and Michael S. Okun.
Published/Produced	New York, NY: Oxford University Press, [2020]
ISBN	9780190647209 (hardback) (epub) (other)
LC classification	RC350.B72 D437 2020
Related names	Chitnis, Shilpa, editor.

Khemani, Pravin, editor.

Okun, Michael S., editor.

Summary

"Tremor is an involuntary movement characterized by a rhythmic oscillation about a fixed point or trajectory. It can be classified based on its clinical features or underlying cause. Tremor was the first approved indication for DBS in the U.S. We now have almost three decades of experience of tremor treatment with DBS. Essential tremor (ET) is the most frequent movement disorder occurring at a frequency of about 5 times that of PD. ET commonly has an autosomal dominant transmission pattern with incomplete penetrance, therefore sporadic cases are not at all uncommon. In ET, most patients suffer from tremor of the hands and arms; approximately 40% suffer from head and 20% from voice tremor. The majority of candidates for functional neurosurgery belong to the ET subgroup which is commonly characterized by severe action or postural tremor that impairs function and quality of life to the extent that the risks, costs and inconvenience of DBS treatment are justified. Unilateral procedures (targeting the thalamus contralateral to the dominant and/or most affected hand) are commonly performed, though bilateral procedures should be considered when limb tremor is severe bilaterally, or when head, voice, or trunk tremors cause significant disability"-- Provided by publisher.

Contents

Introduction to creative programming techniques / Meagen Salinas -- Candidate selection for essential tremor / Laura Surillo Dahdah -- DBS programming for essential tremor / Brent Bluett -

- Utilizing DBS to improve orthostatic tremor / Anhar Hassan -- Bilateral VIM-Thalamic DBS for medication-refractory orthostatic tremor / Mitra Afshari & Jill Ostrem -- Rebound tremor following a sub-optimally placed VIM DBS / Parul Jindal & Joohi Jimenez-Shahed -- Symptomatic cystic lesion following DBS surgery / Vibhash Sharma & Shilpa Chitnis -- Candidate selection for DBS for Parkinson's disease / Laura Surillo Dahdah -- DBS Programming for Parkinson's disease / Raja Mehanna -- Target selection for Parkinson's disease with medication refractory unilateral resting tremor / Fuyuko Sasaki & Genko Oyama -- Genetic mutations and DBS / Jared Hinkle & Zoltan Mari -- Issues to consider when mild cognitive impairment is revealed in pre-operative screening / Sushma Kola & Anhar Hassan -- Use of the STN and GPi deep brain stimulation targets in the same Parkinson's patient: patient specific targeting / Shabbir Hussain I. Merchant & Nora Vanegas-Arroyave -- Medication-refractory Parkinsonian tremor requiring dual lead implantation for tremor control / Anhar Hassan -- Use of constant current mode to allow both monopolar and bipolar interleaving at a single contact / Meredith Spindler & Lana Chahine -- STN-DBS may improve pain in the setting of Parkinson's disease / Anjali Gera, Gian Pal -- DBS responsive camptocormia in Parkinson's disease / Elena Call & Helen Bronte-Stewart -- Deactivation of one STN-DBS device to address brittle ipsilateral dyskinesia in a patient with tremor-dominant Parkinson's disease / Julia Kroth

& Sergiu Groppa -- Management of stimulation-induced dyskinesia in Parkinson disease with interleaving programming settings / Vibhash Sharma & Rajesh Pahwa -- Management of brittle dyskinesia and DDS in subthalamic deep brain stimulation / Junaid Siddiqui & Jawad Bajwa -- Freezing of Gait after Bilateral GPi-DBS in generalized dystonia / Mariana Moskovich -- GPi stimulation-induced gait disturbance and management by re-programming / Dhanya Vijayakumar & Joohi Jimenez-Shahed -- Rescue Vim DBS to address refractory tremor following STN DBS with brittle stimulation-induced dyskinesia / Mitra Afshari & Jill Ostrem -- Postural instability and gait disorder after STN-DBS: Evaluating disease progression, stimulation settings and medication / Javier R. Pérez-Sánchez & Monica M. Kurtis -- Non-surgical management of an exposed DBS lead / Ethan G. Brown & Jill Ostrem -- Steroid-responsive edema interfering with DBS programming / Pravin Khemani & Shilpa Chitnis -- The positive lesion effects of intracranial hemorrhage on DBS surgery outcome / Jacqueline Meystedt & David Charles -- Fibrous scarring and DBS lead implantation / Vinata Vedam Mai & Michael Okun -- Cerebral venous infarction after deep brain stimulation surgery / Andi Nugraha Sendjaja & Takashi Morishita -- Open circuits and loss of DBS benefit in the setting of Parkinson's disease / Arjun Tarakad & Joohi Jimenez-Shahed -- Acute neuropsychiatric symptoms and impulse control disorders after subthalamic nucleus deep brain stimulation / Adolfo Ramirez-Zamora & Michael Okun --

Improved outcome on interleaved deep brain stimulation settings / Svjetlana Miocinovic & Shilpa Chitnis -- Deep brain stimulation targeting the ventral intermediate nucleus of the thalamus for Parkinsonian tremor and later adding the the globus pallidus internus for Parkinson's disease features / Teri Thompsen -- Expected improvement in sleep quality and unexpected improvement in severe nightmares after DBS in Parkinson's disease / Laurice Yang -- Candidate selection for DBS for dystonia / Laura Surillo Dah Dah -- DBS programming for dystonia / Mitesh Lotia -- Choosing a target for DBS in dystonia associated tremor: GPi, VIM, STN, Zi or a combination of targets / Mustafa Siddiqui & Stephen B. Tatter -- Stimulation induced dyskinesia, interleaving settings and management of STN DBS in DYT-1 dystonia / Kyle T. Mitchell & Jill Ostrem -- Deep brain stimulation targeting the globus pallidus internus for dystonic tremor in the setting of generalized dystonia / Teri Thompsen -- Huntington's disease: DBS in adult Huntington's disease for treatment of axial dystonia / Jessica A. Carl and Leo Verhagen Metman -- Aggressiveness: DBS for medically refractory aggressive and injurious behavior / Oscar Bernal-Pacheco -- Bilateral globus pallidus DBS for dystonia and dystonic tremor in spinocerebellar ataxia 17 / Aparna Shukla and Pam Zeilman -- Deep Brain Stimulation for disabling "outflow" tremors: troubleshooting strategies for tremor habituation / Corneliu Luca -- Tardive dystonia and dyskinesia responsive to deep brain stimulation / Irene Malaty.

Subjects	Brain stimulation--Therapeutic use--Case studies.
	Extrapyramidal disorders--Treatment--Case studies.
	Tremor--Treatment--Case studies.
	Nervous system--Surgery--Case studies.
Notes	Includes bibliographical references and index.
Additional formats	Online version: Deep brain stimulation. New York, NY: Oxford University Press, [2020] 9780190647223 (DLC) 2019059949

Diagnostic tests in pediatric pulmonology: applications and interpretation

LCCN	2014951680
Type of material	Book
Main title	Diagnostic tests in pediatric pulmonology: applications and interpretation / Stephanie D. Davis, Ernst Eber, Anastassios C. Koumbourlis, editors.
Published/Produced	New York: Humana Press, [2015]
Description	xi, 321 pages: illustrations; 24 cm
ISBN	9781493918003 (alk. paper)
	1493918001 (alk. paper)
LC classification	RC733 .D465 2015
Related names	Davis, Stephanie D., editor.
	Eber, Ernst, editor.
	Koumbourlis, Anastassios C., editor.
	American Thoracic Society.
Summary	Over the past 20 years, diagnostic tests for pediatric pulmonologists have revolutionized care of children afflicted with respiratory disorders. These tests have been used to not only help in diagnosis, but also in the management and treatment of these children. Bronchoscopic, imaging and physiologic advances have improved

clinical care of these children and have been used as outcome measures in research trials. Diagnostic Tests in Pediatric Pulmonology: Applications and Interpretation describes the various diagnostic modalities (especially the newer ones) that are available for the evaluation of pediatric respiratory disorders. It also provides an understanding of the advantages and limitations of each test so that the clinician may choose the most appropriate ones. An internationally renowned group of authors describe how best to interpret the key findings in a variety of tests as well as the possible pitfalls in incorrect interpretation. This volume focuses on the main diagnostic modalities used in the evaluation of pediatric patients with respiratory disorders and presents up-to-date information on the advantages and limitations of each test for a variety of conditions encountered in the practice of pediatric pulmonology. Clinical utility of these tests is also highlighted. This valuable resource is well suited to practicing clinicians, including pediatric pulmonologists, pediatricians and primary care practitioners, as well as trainees, respiratory therapists and clinical researchers. -- Source other than Library of Congress.

Contents   The Evaluation of the Upper And Lower Airways in Infants and Children.? Principles and Pearls from 4 Decades in the Trenches -- Bronchoalveolar Lavage: Tests and Applications -- Understanding Interventional Bronchoscopy -- Nasal Nitric Oxide and Ciliary Video microscopy: Tests Used for Diagnosing Primary Ciliary Dyskinesia -- Functional Evaluation of Cystic

	Fibrosis Transmembrane Conductance Regulator -- Allergic and Immunologic Testing in Children with Respiratory Disease -- Interpretation of Pulmonary Function Tests in Clinical Practice -- Infant and Preschool Pulmonary Function Tests -- Newer Pulmonary Function Tests -- Selection and Appropriate Use of Spirometric Reference Equations for the Pediatric Population -- Polysomnography for the Pediatric Pulmonologist -- Cardiopulmonary Exercise Testing Techniques to Evaluate Exercise Tolerance -- Imaging for the Pediatric Pulmonologist -- Fractional Exhaled Nitric Oxide: Indications and Interpretation.
Subjects	Medicine.
	Family medicine.
	Critical care medicine.
	Pneumology.
	Pediatrics.
	Child.
	Diagnostic Techniques, Respiratory System.
Notes	Includes bibliographical references and index.
Series	Respiratory medicine; 2197-7372
	Respiratory medicine (New York, N.Y.) 2197-7372

Imaging of the human brain in health and disease

LCCN	2013039184
Type of material	Book
Main title	Imaging of the human brain in health and disease / edited by Philip Seeman, Bertha Madras.
Edition	First edition.
Published/Produced	Amsterdam; Boston: Academic Press/Elsevier, 2014.
Description	xiv, 517 pages: illustrations (some color); 25 cm.

ISBN	9780124186774 (alk. paper)
	0124186777 (alk. paper)
LC classification	RC386.6.T65 I43 2014
Related names	Seeman, Philip, editor of compilation.
	Madras, Bertha, editor of compilation.
Summary	"Modern imaging techniques have allowed researchers to non-invasively peer into the human brain and investigate, among many other things, the acute effects and long-term consequences of drug abuse. Here, we review the most commonly used and some emerging imaging techniques in addiction research, explain how the various techniques generate their characteristic images and describe the rational that researchers use to interpret them. In addition, examples of seminal imaging findings are highlighted that illustrate the contribution of each imaging modality to the expansion in our understanding of the neurobiological bases of drug abuse and addiction, and how they can be parlayed in the future into clinical and therapeutic applications"-- Provided by publisher.
Contents	1. Neuroimaging of Addiction 2. Brain Imaging of Sigma Receptors 3. Imaging of Neurochemical Transmission in the Central Nervous System 4. Human Brain Imaging of Acetylcholine Receptors 5. Human Brain Imaging of Opioid Receptors: Application to CNS Biomarker and Drug Development 6. Human Brain Imaging of Adenosine Receptors 7. Human Brain Imaging of Dopamine D1 Receptors 8. Human Brain Imaging of Dopamine Transporters 9. Dopamine Receptor Imaging in Schizophrenia: Focus on Genetic Vulnerability 10. Human Brain Imaging of Anger

	11. Imaging Pain in the Human Brain 12. Imaging of Dopamine and Serotonin Receptors and Transporters 13. Imaging the Dopamine D3 Receptor In Vivo 14. Human Brain Imaging of Autism Spectrum Disorders 15. Brain PET Imaging in the Cannabinoid System 16. Brain Imaging of Cannabinoid Receptors 17. Human Brain Imaging In Tardive Dyskinesia 18. Dopamine Receptors and Dopamine Release 19. Radiotracers Used to Image the Brains of Patients with Alzheimer's Disease.
Subjects	Brain--Tomography.
	Brain--Diseases--Diagnosis.
	Neuroimaging--methods.
	Brain Chemistry--physiology.
	Brain Diseases--radionuclide imaging.
	Mental Disorders--radionuclide imaging.
	Substance-Related Disorders--radionuclide imaging.
Notes	Includes bibliographical references and index.
Series	Neuroscience-net reference book series; book 1

Involuntary movements: classification and video atlas

LCCN	2019031816
Type of material	Book
Personal name	Shibasaki, Hiroshi, 1939- author.
Main title	Involuntary movements: classification and video atlas / Hiroshi Shibasaki, Mark Hallett, Stephen G. Reich, Kailash P. Bhatia; associate author, Bettina Balint.
Published/Produced	New York, NY: Oxford University Press, [2020]
Description	1 online resource
ISBN	9780190865078 (card)
	9780190865054 (online)

	9780190865061 (online)
	(hardback)
LC classification	RC394.T37
Related names	Hallett, Mark, 1943- author.
	Reich, Stephen G., author.
	Bhatia, Kailash, author.
	Balint, Bettina, author.
Summary	"This book is aimed at describing clinical features of various kinds of involuntary movements by demonstrating a number of cases on video. All cases presented in this book were directly observed and studied by at least one of the five authors. We will also discuss the current consensus about the classification, pathophysiology and current treatment of each involuntary movement. This book adopts a unique way of looking at movement disorders; that is considering two aspects of the diagnosis, axis 1, the phenomenology and, axis 2, the etiology and/or pathophysiology. The visual appearance (video) is a big part of axis 1"-- Provided by publisher.
Contents	Definition and classification of involuntary movements -- Tremor -- Myoclonus -- Chorea and ballism -- Athetosis and dystonia -- Dyskinesia, motor stereotypies and tics -- Functional movement disorders (psychogenic involuntary movements) -- Sleep-related movement disorders -- Disorders of increased muscle stiffness or overactivity.
Subjects	Dyskinesias--physiopathology
	Dyskinesias--classification
Notes	Includes bibliographical references and index.

Involuntary movements: classification and video atlas

LCCN	2019031815
Type of material	Book
Personal name	Shibasaki, Hiroshi, 1939- author.
Main title	Involuntary movements: classification and video atlas / Hiroshi Shibasaki, Mark Hallett, Kailash P. Bhatia, Stephen G. Reich; associate author, Bettina Balint.
Published/Produced	New York, NY: Oxford University Press, [2020]
Description	xvii, 190 pages: illustrations; 25 cm
ISBN	9780190865047 (hardback)
	(online)
	(online)
	(card)
LC classification	RC394.T37 S53 2020
Related names	Hallett, Mark, 1943- author.
	Bhatia, Kailash, author.
	Reich, Stephen G., author.
	Balint, Bettina, author.
Summary	"This book is aimed at describing clinical features of various kinds of involuntary movements by demonstrating a number of cases on video. All cases presented in this book were directly observed and studied by at least one of the five authors. We will also discuss the current consensus about the classification, pathophysiology and current treatment of each involuntary movement. This book adopts a unique way of looking at movement disorders; that is considering two aspects of the diagnosis, axis 1, the phenomenology and, axis 2, the etiology and/or pathophysiology. The visual appearance (video) is a big part of axis 1"-- Provided by publisher.

Contents	Definition and classification of involuntary movements -- Tremor -- Myoclonus -- Chorea and ballism -- Athetosis and dystonia -- Dyskinesia, motor stereotypies and tics -- Functional movement disorders (psychogenic involuntary movements) -- Sleep-related movement disorders -- Disorders of increased muscle stiffness or overactivity.
Subjects	Tardive dyskinesia. Dyskinesias--physiopathology Dyskinesias--classification
Notes	Includes bibliographical references and index.

Levodopa-induced dyskinesia in Parkinson's disease

LCCN	2014951222
Type of material	Book
Main title	Levodopa-induced dyskinesia in Parkinson's disease / [edited by] Susan H. Fox.
Published/Produced	New York: Springer, 2014.
ISBN	9781447165026 (hard cover: alk. paper)

Marsden's book of movement disorders

LCCN	2012471553
Type of material	Book
Main title	Marsden's book of movement disorders / Ivan Donaldson ... [et al.].
Published/Created	Oxford: Oxford University Press, 2012.
Description	xiv, 1497 p.: ill., ports.; 28 cm.
ISBN	9780192619112 (alk. paper) 019261911X (alk. paper)
LC classification	RC376.5 .M37 2012
Variant title	Book of movement disorders
Portion of title	Movement disorders
Related names	Marsden, C. David.

Contents

Donaldson, Ivan.
Sect. 1. Structure and function of the basal ganglia. Anatomy functions of the basal ganglia -- Sect. 2. Clinical approach to movement disorders. Clinical assessment -- Investigation -- Sect. 3. Akinetic-rigid syndromes. Introduction -- Sect. 3A. Idiopathic/primary syndromes. Parkinson's disease -- Multiple system atrophy -- Progressive supranuclear palsy (or Steele-Richardson-Olszewski disease) -- Corticobasal degeneration -- Parkinsonian-dementia syndromes -- Sect. 3B. Symptomatic parkinsonian syndromes inherited. Wilson's disease -- Pantothenate kinase-associated neurodegeneration (PKAN), previously also known as Hallervorden-Spatz disease -- Sect. 3C. Symptomatic parkinsonian syndromes acquired. Postencephalic parkinsonism -- Drug-induced parkinsonism and the neuroleptic malignant syndrome -- Basal ganglia calcification -- Other acquired symptomatic parkinsonian syndromes -- Sect. 4. Tremor. Introduction. Physiological and exaggerated or enhanced physiological tremor -- Classical essential tremor -- Isolated site-specific or task-specific tremors -- Symptomatic tremors -- Sect. 5. Chorea. Introduction. Sect. 5A. Idiopathic choreic syndromes. Huntington's disease -- Other idiopathic choreic syndromes -- Sect. 5B. Symptomatic choreic syndromes. Sydenham's chorea -- Spontaneous oro-facial chorea and tardive dyskinesia -- Other symptomatic (secondary) choreic syndromes -- Ballism -- Sect. 6. Tics. Introduction. Sect. 6A. Idiopathic (primary) tic syndromes. Simple tics --

	Gilles de la Tourette's syndrome -- Symptomatic (secondary) tic syndromes -- Sect. 7. Myoclonus. Focal myoclonus -- Epileptic myoclonus -- Brainstem myoclonus and startle syndromes -- Specific myoclonic syndromes -- Other specific causes of symptomatic generalized myoclonus -- Essential myoclonus -- Sect. 8. Dystonia. Introduction. Sect. 8A. Primary (idiopathic) dystonic syndromes. Generalized primary dystonia -- Other primary dystonias (dystonia-plus syndromes) -- Idiopathic (primary) cranial dystonias -- Spasmodic torticollis -- Writer's and craft cramps -- Sect. 8B. Secondary (symptomatic) dystonic syndromes. Lesch-Nyhan syndrome -- Other inherited secondary (symptomatic) dystonias -- Cerebral palsy -- Other acquired secondary (symptomatic) dystonic syndromes -- Sect. 9. Syndromes of continuous muscle fibre activity. Introduction. Stiff man syndromes -- Neuromyotonic syndromes -- Sect. 10. Restlessness. Introduction. Akathisia -- Restless legs syndrome -- Painful legs and moving toes -- Sect. 11. Episodic movement disorders. Introduction. Paroxysmal choreic, athetotic, or dystonic attacks -- Tonic attacks -- Intermittent ataxias -- Sect. 12. Miscellaneous movement disorders. Miscellaneous movement disorders.
Subjects	Movement disorders. Movement Disorders.
Notes	Includes bibliographical references and index.

Medaka: a model for organogenesis, human disease, and evolution

LCCN	2011925865
Type of material	Book

Main title	Medaka: a model for organogenesis, human disease, and evolution / Kiyoshi Naruse, Minoru Tanaka, Hiroyuki Takeda, editors.
Published/Created	Tokyo; New York: Springer, c2011.
Description	xvii, 387 p.: ill.; 25 cm.
ISBN	9784431926900 (alk. paper)
	4431926909 (alk. paper)
	9784431926917 (e-ISBN)
	4431926917 (e-ISBN)
LC classification	QL638.O78 M426 2011
Related names	Naruse, Kiyoshi, Ph. D.
	Tanaka, Minoru, 1961-
	Takeda, Hiroyuki, 1958-
Contents	A glance at the past of medaka fish biology / Hiroshi Hori -- Genetics, genomics, and biological resources in the medaka, Oryzias latipes / Kiyoshi Naruse -- Chromatin-associated periodicity in genetic variation downstream of transcriptional start sites / Shin Sasaki ... [et al.] -- Transposable elements Tol1 and Tol2 / Akihiko Koga -- A systematic screen for mutations affecting organogenesis in medaka / Makoto Furutani-Seiki -- Medaka bone development / Akira Kudo -- Anatomical atlas of blood vascular system of medaka / Sumio Isogai and Misato Fujita -- Kidney development, regeneration, and polycystic kidney disease in medaka / Hisashi Hashimoto -- Primary ciliary dyskinesia in fish: the analysis of a novel medaka mutant kintoun / Daisuke Kobayashi and Hiroyuki Takeda -- p53-deficient medaka created by TILLING / Yoshihito Taniguchi -- Medaka spontaneous mutants for body coloration / Shoji Fukamachi -- Craniofacial traits / Minori Shinya -- Double anal fin (Da): a

medaka mutant exhibiting a mirror-image pattern duplication of the dorsal-ventral axis / Masato Ohtsuka, Hiroyuki Takeda, and Atsuko Shimada -- Interaction of germ cells and gonadal somatic cells during gonadal formation / Minoru Tanaka -- Frequent turnover of sex chromosomes in the medaka fishes / Yusuke Takehana -- Function of the medaka male sex-determining gene / Manfred Schartl -- The sex-determining gene in medaka / Masaru Matsuda -- Endocrine regulation of oogenesis in the medaka, Oryzias latipes / Naoki Shibata ... [et al.] -- Interspecific medaka hybrids as experimental models for investigating cell division and germ cell development / Toshiharu Iwai ... [et al.] -- Reconstruction of the vertebrate ancestral genome reveals dynamic genome reorganization in early vertebrates / Yoichiro Nakatani ... [et al.] -- Genome duplication and subfunction partitioning: Sox9 in medaka and other vertebrates / Hayato Yokoi and John H. Postlethwait -- Human population genetics meets medaka / Hiroki Oota and Hiroshi Mitani -- Evolution of the major histocompatibility complex: a lesson from the Oryzias species / Masaru Nonaka and Kentaro Tsukamoto -- Molecular evolution of teleostean hatching enzymes and their egg envelope digestion mechanism: an aspect of co-evolution of protease and substrate / Shigeki Yasumasu, Kaori Sano, and Mari Kawaguchi.

Subjects Oryzias latipes.
Oryzias latipes--Genetics.
Oryzias latipes--Functional genomics.
Diseases--Animal models.

	Fish as laboratory animals.
	Animals, Laboratory.
	Oryzias--genetics.
	Disease Models, Animal.
	Evolution, Molecular.
	Organogenesis--genetics.
Notes	Includes bibliographical references and index.

Merritt's neurology.

LCCN	2009033401
Type of material	Book
Main title	Merritt's neurology.
Edition	12th ed. / editors, Lewis P. Rowland, Timothy A. Pedley.
Published/Created	Philadelphia, PA: Lippincott Williams & Wilkins, c2010.
Description	xxi, 1172 p.: ill.; 29 cm.
Links	Publisher description http://www.loc.gov/catdir/enhancements/fy0917/2009033401-d.html
	Table of contents only http://www.loc.gov/catdir/enhancements/fy1012/2009033401-t.html
ISBN	9780781791861
	0781791863
LC classification	RC346 .M4 2010
Portion of title	Neurology
Related names	Rowland, Lewis P.
	Pedley, Timothy A.
	Merritt, H. Houston (Hiram Houston), 1902-1979.
Contents	Signs and symptoms in neurologic diagnosis: approach to the patient -- Delirium and confusion -- Memory loss, behavioral changes and dementia -- Aphasia, apraxia, and agnosia -- Syncope, seizures and their mimics -- Coma -- Headache --

Diagnosis of pain and paresthesias -- Dizziness, vertigo, and hearing loss -- Impaired vision -- Involuntary movements -- Syndromes caused by weak muscles -- Gait disorders -- CT and MRI -- Electroencephalography and evoked potentials -- Electromyography, nerve conduction studies, and and magnetic stimulation -- Autonomic testing -- Neurovascular imaging -- Endovascular neuroradiology -- Lumbar puncture and cerebrospinal fluid examination -- Muscle and nerve biopsy -- Neuropsychological evaluation -- DNA diagnosis -- Bacterial infections -- Focal infections -- Viral infections and postviral syndromes -- Human immunodeficiency virus (HIV) and acquired immunodeficiency syndrome (AIDS) -- Fungal infections -- Neurosarcoidosis -- Neurosyphilis -- Leptospirosis -- Lyme disease -- Parasitic infections -- Bacterial toxins -- Prion diseases -- Whipple disease -- Pathogenesis, classification, and epidemiology of cerebrovascular disease -- Examination of the patient with cerebrovascular disease -- Transient ischemic attack -- Cerebral infarction -- Intracerebral hemorrhage -- Genetics of stroke -- Other cerebrovascular syndromes -- Differential diagnosis of stroke -- Stroke in children -- Treatment and prevention of stroke -- Subarachnoid hemorrhage -- Cerebral venous and sinus thrombosis -- Vascular disease of the spinal cord -- Vasculitis -- Susac syndrome -- Vascular tumors and malformations -- Hydrocephalus -- Normal pressure hydrocephalus (NPH) -- Brain edema and disorders of intracranial pressure -- Superficial siderosis and intracerebral hypotension -- Hyperosmolar syndromes -- General considerations -- Tumors of the skull and cranial nerves -- Tumors of the meninges -- Gliomas -- Lymphomas -- Pineal region tumors -- Tumors of the pituitary gland -- Congenital and childhood tumors -- Metastatic tumors -- Spinal tumors -- Paraneoplastic syndromes -- Complications of cancer chemotherapy -- Head injury -- Spine injury -- Cranial and peripheral nerve lesions -- Complex regional pain syndrome -- Radiation injury -- Electrical and lightning injury -- Decompression sickness -- Intervertebral dics and radiculopathy -- Cervical spondylotic myelopathy -- Thoracic outlet syndrome -- Hereditary and acquired spastic paraplegia -- Syringomyelia -- Neonatal neurology -- Floppy infant syndrome -- Disorders of motor and mental development -- Autism spectrum disorders -- Laurence-Moon-Biedl syndrome -- Cerebral and spinal malformations -- Chromosomal diseases -- Marcus Gunn -- Möbius syndrome -- Disorders of amino acid metabolism -- Disorders of purine and pyrimidine metabolism -- Lysosomal and other storage diseases -- Disorders of carbohydrate metabolism -- Glucose transporter type 1 deficiency syndrome -- Disorders of DNA maintenance, transcription, and translation -- Hyperammonemia -- Peroxisomal diseases: adrenoleukodystrophy, zellweger syndrome, and refsum disease -- Organic acidurias -- Disorders of metal metabolism -- Acute intermittent porphyria -- Neurologic syndromes with acanthocytes -- Cerebral degenerations of childhood -- Diffuse sclerosis and vanishing white matter disease -- Mitochondrial encephalomyopathies: diseases of mitochondrial DNA -- Leber hereditary optic neuropathy -- Mitochondrial diseases with mutations of nuclear DNA -- Neurofibromatosis -- Tuberous sclerosis complex -- Encephalotrigeminal angiomatosis -- Incontinentia pigmenti -- General considerations -- Alzheimer disease -- Frontotemporal dementia -- Lewy body dementias -- Huntington disease -- Choreas -- Myoclonus -- Gilles de la tourette syndrome -- Dystonia -- Essential tremor -- Parkinson disease -- Parkinson-plus syndromes -- Paroxysmal dyskinesias -- Tradive dyskinesia and other neuroleptic-induced syndromes -- Autosomal recessive ataxias -- Autosomal dominant ataxias -- Amyotrophic lateral sclerosis, progressive muscular atrophy, and primary lateral sclerosis -- Kennedy disease -- Spinal muscular atrophies of childhood -- Monomelic muscular atrophy -- General considerations -- The inherited peripheral neuropathies -- Acquired neuropathies -- Neuropathic pain -- Myasthenia gravis -- Lambert-Eaton syndrome -- Botulism and antibiotic-induced neuromuscular disorders -- Critical illness myopathy and neuropathy -- Identifying disorders of the motor unit -- Progressive muscular dystrophies -- Familial periodic paralysis -- Congenital disorders of muslce -- Myoglobinuria -- Muscle cramps and stiffness -- Dermatomyositis -- Polymyositis, inclusion body myositis, and related myopathies -- Myositis ossificans -- Multiple sclerosis -- Neuromyelitis optica -- Marchiafava-Bignami disease -- Central pontine myelinolysis --

Epilepsy -- Febrile seizures -- Primary and secondary headaches -- Transient global amnesia -- Ménière syndrome -- Sleep disorders -- Neurogenic orthostatic hypotension, autonomic failure, and autonomic neuropathy -- Familial dysautonomia -- Endocrine diseases -- Hematologic and related diseases -- Hepatic disease -- Cerebral complications of cardiac surgery -- Bone disease -- Renal disease -- Respiratory support for neurologic diseases -- Nutritional disorders: malnutrition, malabsorption, and B_{12} and other vitamin deficiency -- Hypertrophic pachymeningitis -- Neurologic disease during pregnancy -- Hashimoto encephalopathy -- Schizophrenia -- Mood disorders -- Anxiety disorders -- Somatoform disorders -- Alcoholism -- Drug dependence -- Iatrogenic disease -- Occupational and environmental neurotoxicology -- HIV, fetal alcohol and drug effects, and the battered child -- Falls in the elderly -- Neurologic rehabilitation -- End-of-life issues in neurology.

Subjects	Nervous system--Diseases.
	Neurology.
	Nervous System Diseases.
Notes	Includes bibliographical references and index.

Nursing care in pediatric respiratory disease

LCCN	2011021938
Type of material	Book
Main title	Nursing care in pediatric respiratory disease / edited by Concettina (Tina) Tolomeo.
Edition	1st ed.

Published/Created	Chichester, West Sussex; Ames, Iowa: John Wiley & Sons, 2012.
Description	xvii, 338 p.: ill.; 25 cm.
ISBN	9780813817682 (pbk.: alk. paper)
	0813817684 (pbk.: alk. paper)
	9780470962947 (ePDF)
	0470962941 (ePDF)
	9780470962978 (ePub)
	0470962976 (ePub)
	9780470963005 (Mobi)
	047096300X (Mobi)
LC classification	RJ431 .N87 2012
Related names	Tolomeo, Concettina.
Contents	Pediatric pulmonary anatomy and physiology / Neal Nakra -- Pediatric respiratory health history and physical assessment / Concettina Tolomeo -- Principles of lung therapeutics / Kathryn Blake -- Neonatal lung disease: apnea of prematurity and bronchopulmonary dysplasia / Pnina Weiss and Concettina Tolomeo -- Lower airway disease / Julie Honey and Michael Bye -- Upper airway disorders / Wendy S.L. Mackey, Melissa M. Dziedzic, and Lisa M. Gagnon -- Asthma / Concettina Tolomeo, Dawn Baker, and Pnina Weiss -- Cystic fibrosis / Antoinette Gardner and Kimberly Jones -- Obstructive sleep apnea / Linda Niemiec and Lewis J. Kass -- Primary ciliary dyskinesia and bronchiectasis / Rosalyn Bravo and Anita Bhandari -- Acute respiratory problems / Marcia Winston and Catherine Kier.
Subjects	Pediatric respiratory diseases--Nursing.
	Respiratory Tract Diseases--nursing.
	Child.
	Pediatric Nursing--methods.

Notes	Includes bibliographical references and index.

Psychiatric disorders: methods and protocols
LCCN	2011943889
Type of material	Book
Main title	Psychiatric disorders: methods and protocols / edited by Firas H. Kobeissy.
Published/Created	New York: Humana Press, c2012.
Description	xxi, 610 p.: ill. 27 cm.
Links	http://digitool.hbz-nrw.de:1801/webclient/DeliveryManager?pid=4406683&custom_att_2=simple_viewer Psychiatric disorders
ISBN	9781617794575 (alk. paper)
	1617794570 (alk. paper)
	9781617794582 (e-ISBN)
LC classification	RC454 .P769 2012
Related names	Kobeissy, Firas H. edt
Contents	New frontiers in animal research of psychiatric illness / Arie Kaffman and John J. Krystal -- Experimental psychiatric illness and drug abuse models: from human to animal, an overview / Scott Edwards and George F. Koob -- Qualitative versus quantitative methods in psychiatric research / Mahdi Razafsha ... [et al.] -- Animal models of self-injurious behaviour: an overview / Darragh P. Devine -- Rodent models of adaptive decision making / Alicia Izquierdo and Annabelle M. Belcher -- Animal models of depression and neuroplasticity: assessing drug action in relation to behavior and neurogenesis / Ying Xu ... [et al.] -- Modeling depression in animal models / David H. Overstreet -- Behavioral model for assessing cognitive decline / Michael Guidi and Thomas C.

Foster -- The pemoline model of self-injurious behaviour / Darraugh P. Devine -- Modeling risky decision making in rodents / Nicholas W. Simon and Barry Setlow -- Open space anxiety test in rodents: the elevated platform with steep slopes / Abdelkader Ennaceur -- An animal model to study the molecular basis of tardive dyskinesia / Mahendra Bishnoi and Ravneet K. Boparai -- Models of chronic alcohol exposure and dependence / darin J. Knapp and George R. Breese -- Rat models of prenatal and adolescent cannabis exposure / Jennifer A. DiNieri and Yasmin L. Hurd -- Modeling nicotine addiction in rats / Stephanie Caille ... [et al.] -- Animal models of nicotine withdrawal: intracranial self-stimulation and somatic signs of withdrawal / Rayna M. Bauzo and Adrie W. Bruijnzeel -- Methods in drug abuse models: comparison of different models of methamphetamine paradigms / Firas H. Kobeissy ... [et al.] -- Cocaine self-administration in rats: hold-down procedures / Benjamin A. Zimmer and David C.S. Roberts -- Cocaine self-administration in rats: discrete trials procedures / Carson V. Dobrin and David C.S. Roberts -- Cocaine self-administration in rats: threshold procedures / Erik B. Oleson and David C.S. Roberts -- Assessing locomotor-stimulating effects of cocaine in rodents / Drake Morgan ... [et al.] -- Methods in tobacco abuse: proteomic changes following second-hand smoke exposure / Joy Guingab-Cagmat ... [et al.] -- Animal models of sugar and fat bingeing: relationship to food addiction and increased body weight / Nicole M. Avena, Miriam E. Bocarsly, and Bartley G.

Hoebel -- Animal models of overeating / Neil E. Rowland -- The activity-based anorexia mouse model / Stephanie J. Klenotich and Stephanie C. Dulawa -- Dissociating behavioral, autonomic, and neuroendocrine effects of androgen steroids in animal models / Amy S. Kohtz and Cheryl A. Frye -- Interleukin-2 and the septohippocampal system: intrinsic actions and autoimmune processes relevant to neuropsychiatric disorders / John M. Petitto ... [et al.] -- Experimental schizophrenia models in rodents established with inflammatory agents and cytokines / Hiroyuki Nawa and Kiyofumi Yamada -- P11: a potential biomarker for posttraumatic stress disorder / Lei Zhang, Robert J. Ursano, and He Li -- Investigation of age-specific behavioral and proteomic changes in an animal model of chronic ethanol exposure / Antoinette M. Maldonado-Devincci, Stanley M. Stevens Jr., and Cheryl L. Kirstein -- Quantitative peptidomics to measure neuropeptide levels in animal models relevant to psychiatric disorders / Julia S. Gelman ... [et al.] -- ADHD animal model characterization: transcriptomics and proteomics analyses / Yoshinori Masuo, Junko Shibato, and Randeep Rakwal -- Psychiatric disorder biomarker discovery using quantitative proteomics / Michaela D. Filiou and Christoph W. Turck -- Gene profiling of laser-microdissected brain regions and individual cells in drug abuse and schizophrenia research / Pietro Paolo Sanna, Vez Repunte-Canonigo, and Alessandro Guidotti -- Stable isotope labeling with amino acids in cell culture-based proteomic analysis of ethanol-

	induced protein expression profiles in microglia / Bin Liu, David S. Barber, and Stanley M. Stevens Jr. -- Systems biology in psychiatric research: from complex data sets over wiring diagrams to computer simulations / Felix Tretter and Peter J. Gebicke-Haerter -- Data mining in psychiatric research / Diego Tovar ... [et al.]
Subjects	Mental illness--Laboratory manuals.
	Mental Disorders--Laboratory Manuals.
	Substance-Related Disorders--Laboratory Manuals.
	Animal Experimentation--Laboratory Manuals.
	Animals, Laboratory.
Notes	Includes bibliographical references and index.
Series	Methods in molecular biology; 829
	Springer protocols
	Methods in molecular biology (Clifton, N.J.); v. 829. 1064-3745
	Springer protocols.

Tardive dyskinesia: current approach

LCCN	2018946230
Type of material	Book
Main title	Tardive dyskinesia: current approach / Chanoch Miodownik and Vladimir Lerner, editors.
Published/Produced	New York: Nova Medicine & Health, [2018]
Description	viii, 195 pages; 23 cm.
ISBN	9781536137767 (pbk.)
	1536137766 (pbk.)
LC classification	MLCM 2018/48273 (R)
Related names	Miodownik, Chanoch, editor.
	Lerner, Vladimir, editor.
Subjects	Tardive dyskinesia.
Notes	Includes bibliographical references and index.

Series	Rare disorders research progress

Video protocols and techniques for movement disorders

LCCN	2015013965
Type of material	Book
Personal name	Barton, Brandon R., author.
Main title	Video protocols and techniques for movement disorders / Brandon R. Barton, Deborah A. Hall.
Published/Produced	Oxford; New York: Oxford University Press, [2016]
ISBN	9780199948512 (alk. paper)
LC classification	RC376.5
Related names	Hall, Deborah A., author.
Contents	Technical aspects of videotaping -- Environment for taping -- Consent issues for videotaping -- Instructions for the videographer -- Editing videos for publication -- General -- Parkinson disease -- Atypical Parkinsonian disorders -- Deep brain stimulator surgery evaluation -- Dyskinesia -- Tremor -- Dystonia -- Ataxia -- Tics and Tourette syndrome -- Chorea -- Myoclonus -- Functional movement disorders.
Subjects	Movement Disorders--diagnosis. Neurologic Examination--methods. Video Recording--methods.
Notes	Includes bibliographical references and index.

Related Nova Publications

Tardive Dyskinesia: Current Approach

Chanoch Miodownik, M.D.
and Vladimir Lerner, M.D., Ph.D. (Editors)
Ben-Gurion University of the Negev, Be'er Sheva, Israel

ISBN: 978-1-53613-777-4
Binding: Softcover
Publication Date: August 2018

Abnormal involuntary dyskinetic movements in schizophrenia patients have been documented for more than 140 years. However, after introducing into clinical practice antipsychotic medications, movement disturbances became a relatively frequent phenomenon. Medication-induced movement disorders are divided into two groups: a) acute, which appears during several hours or days after beginning treatment with psychotropic medications, and b) delayed or tardive motor disturbances that occur after months or years of taking psychotropic drugs. In the term's present meaning, the latter are iatrogenic, neurological, hyperkinetic movement disturbances characterized by repetitive, involuntary, purposeless movements in the oral/lingual/buccal area, body or choreoathetoid movements of the extremities.

Tardive movement disorder (TMD) is a serious, disabling and potentially permanent pathology. The pathogenesis of TMD remains unclear, and the pathophysiology is complex, multifactorial, and still not fully understood. Moreover, there is solid evidence of a genetic predisposition to these disturbances.

Abnormal movements should appear during exposure, or within four weeks of withdrawal from oral psychotropic medications or eight weeks from depot formulations. The minimal exposure to these drugs should be three months, except for patients older than 60, who can develop TMD after its use for one month. Finally, the movements should be present for at least one month to fulfill the criteria for TMD.

Several distinct forms of TMD exist, specifically tardive akathisia, tardive blepharospasm, tardive dystonia, tardive gait, tardive myoclonus, tardive tremor, and tardive tics, and they have different pathophysiologies and treatment.

The advent and widespread use of a new generation of antipsychotics in clinical practice had been expected to dramatically reduce the incidence and prevalence of TMD, however the reduction, if any, was modest. A number of drugs were tried for the management of this motor disturbance, yet until now no effective and standard treatment has been found. Therefore, the management of this motor disturbance remains an actual topic as well as a challenge for clinicians.

Although much has been written about TMD, this is obviously not a new clinical issue. Awareness of these motor disturbances as a result of medication treatment is a vital step toward intervention in the pathological process. Furthermore, it will be helpful for the protection and prevention of serious complications, while also allowing for greater access to clinicians in overall areas of medicine.

The authors believe that a better understanding of TMD will strengthen the efforts and success of effective diagnosing, prevention and treatment of this condition.

PRIMARY CILIARY DYSKINESIA[*]

Rheanne Maravelas[†], MD and
Myrtha Gregoire-Bottex, MD
Departments of Internal Medicine,
Department of Pediatric and Adolescent Medicine,
Western Michigan University Homer Stryker MD School of Medicine,
Kalamazoo, Michigan, USA

Primary ciliary dyskinesia is a chronic disease of the respiratory tract that involves defects of cilia that are found in various structures such as the respiratory tract, fallopian tube and sperm cell flagella. This discussion considers various aspects of this disorder, including its pathophysiology, diagnosis, management and prognosis. Also considered are extra-pulmonary features and genetic principles found in this disorder.

---

[*] The full version of this chapter can be found in *Chronic Disease and Disability: The Pediatric Lung*, edited by Donald E Greydanus, M.D., Myrtha M Gregoire-Bottex, M.D., Kevin W Cates and Joav Merrick, M.D., published by Nova Science Publishers, Inc, New York, 2018.
[†] Correspondence: Rheanne Maravelas, MD, Departments of Internal Medicine, Pediatric and Adolescent Medicine, Western Michigan University Homer Stryker MD School of Medicine, 1000 Oakland Drive, Kalamazoo, MI 49008, United States. Email: Rheanne.maravelas@ med.wmich.edu.

PRIMARY CILIARY DYSKINESIA – CURRENT THERAPEUTIC APPROACH[*]

Peter Durdik[†] *and Peter Banovcin*

Department of Pediatrics,
Center of Experimental and Clinical Respirology,
Comenius University Jessenius Faculty of Medicine, Martin, Slovakia

Primary ciliary dyskinesia is a rare heterogeneous genetic disorder with an incidence estimated to be between 1:2000 and 1:40000. Over 250 proteins are involved in the formation of cilia and to date, the twenty-six genes have been identified in association with primary ciliary dyskinesia. However, despite the various genotypes that can cause primary ciliary dyskinesia, the clinical phenotypes are very similar. Affected ciliary function is characterized by ciliary immotility or dysmotility, impairing mucociliary clearance which is responsible for typical clinical symptoms (chronic recurrent upper and lower respiratory tract infections, male sterility and situs inversus in 40% - 50% of patients). Early diagnosis is essential to ensure specialist management and to reduce respiratory and ontological complications. The diagnosis of primary ciliary dyskinesia should be established on the presence of the characteristic clinical phenotype, appropriate screening tests, specific ultrastructural ciliary defects, evidence of abnormal ciliary function and genetic analysis. There is currently no specific pharmacological, non-pharmacological or surgical treatment that restores normal ciliary motility and improves mucus clearance. All treatment recommendations are based on very low level evidence. The guidelines for

---

[*] The full version of this chapter can be found in *Advances in Respiratory Therapy Research*, edited by Miloš Jeseňák., published by Nova Science Publishers, Inc, New York, 2014.
[†] Corresponding Author address: Peter Durdik, M.D., Ph.D., Department of Pediatris, Center of Experimental and Clinical Respirology, Jessenius Faculty of Medicine in Martin, Comenius University in Bratislava, University Hospital, Kollarova 2, 036 59, Martin, Slovak Republic, e-mail: Peter.Durdik@jfmed.uniba.sk

the management of primary ciliary dyskinesia in children, published by the ERS PCD Task Force in 2009, present the treatment based on periodic monitoring of the general condition, respiratory and auditory function, promotion of drainage of secretions through respiratory physiotherapy and physical exercise and aggressive antibiotic treatment of respiratory infections. The curative treatment of primary ciliary dyskinesia is still unavailable, although gene therapy has major potential for treating ciliopathies. Other recently presented positive therapeutic modalities include alpha-1-antitrypsin, antiprotease and secretory immunoglobulin A.

TARDIVE DYSKINESIA[*]

Nisha Warikoo[1], Thomas L. Schwartz[1,†] and Leslie Citrome[2]

[1]SUNY Upstate Medical University,
Department of Psychiatry, Syracuse, NY, US
[2]New York Medical College, Valhalla, NY, US

Introduction: The treatment of schizophrenia was revolutionized by the introduction of first-generation antipsychotics (FGAs) in the 1950s. FGAs have now been largely replaced by second-generation antipsychotics (SGAs), which have a lower propensity for acute extrapyramidal symptoms (EPS)[1,2] and perhaps tardive dyskinesia (TD).[3] There remains a need however to be able to accurately detect and manage motoric side effects of antipsychotics as these problems persist in clinical practice.

Conclusion: Tardive dyskinesia rates appear to be lower with newer antipsychotic agents but still a problematic side effect that requires astute

---

[*] The full version of this chapter can be found in *Antipsychotic Drugs: Pharmacology, Side Effects and Abuse Prevention*, edited by Thomas L. Schwartz, James Megna and Michael E. Topel., published by Nova Science Publishers, Inc, New York, 2012.
[†] Tel:315 464-3100. FAX:315 464-3163. E-mail:schwartt@upstate.edu.

clinical skills for detection and mitigation. This chapter will review all aspects of this side effect to aid clinicians' ability to provide safe patient care while prescribing second generation antipsychotics.

INDEX

A

abnormal involuntary movement (AIM), viii, 90, 103, 104, 108, 109, 111
abuse, 97, 158, 174
acid, 85, 90, 100, 112
activities of daily living (ADL), 107
adaptation(s), vii, ix, 51, 103, 108
adulthood, 8, 11, 17, 18, 21, 48, 49
adults, 7, 8, 9, 10, 12, 16, 17, 18, 19, 49, 51, 114, 115
adverse effects, 86, 89, 133
age, 5, 6, 8, 10, 11, 12, 15, 26, 38, 49, 51, 54, 55, 71, 72, 73, 115, 175
airway inflammation, 52, 55, 60
airways, vii, 2, 4, 11, 18, 20, 30, 49, 59, 144, 145
akathisia, 74, 83, 84, 114, 132, 180
ALI, 44, 45, 46, 47
amino, 107, 169, 175
amino acid, 107, 169, 175
amplitude, 28, 32, 33, 77
antibiotic, 6, 14, 18, 27, 170, 183
antipsychotic, 91, 92, 105, 111, 131, 138, 179, 183

anxiety, 88, 137, 174
assessment, viii, 20, 44, 69, 163, 172
ataxia, 106, 118, 140, 142, 150, 154
atelectasis, 11, 15, 49
athetosis, viii, 103, 117
autosomal dominant, 117, 146, 151
autosomal recessive, viii, 2, 31, 48

B

bacteria, vii, 2, 10
basal ganglia, 76, 77, 80, 81, 163
bilateral, 86, 147, 151
biopsy, 39, 46, 47, 144
brain, 14, 81, 87, 94, 133, 134, 146, 148, 150, 153, 155, 175, 177
breathing, 26, 70, 116
bronchiectasis, 4, 6, 7, 11, 15, 16, 17, 18, 21, 26, 35, 49, 53, 59, 60, 145, 172
bronchitis, 4, 6, 145

C

cell culture, 19, 21, 24, 28, 39, 43, 44, 45, 46, 47, 62, 67, 68, 175

childhood, 6, 7, 17, 49, 54, 60, 169
children, 5, 6, 7, 8, 10, 12, 18, 19, 20, 25, 51, 52, 54, 55, 56, 57, 59, 60, 61, 62, 64, 96, 155, 168, 183
chorea, viii, 94, 103, 104, 105, 114, 118, 134, 140, 142, 163
cilia, vii, 2, 3, 4, 6, 7, 13, 21, 24, 27, 28, 29, 30, 31, 32, 33, 34, 38, 39, 40, 41, 42, 43, 44, 45, 46, 47, 48, 49, 50, 53, 57, 61, 62, 63, 64, 65, 181, 182
cilia structure and function, 3
classification, 117, 131, 133, 136, 139, 143, 146, 150, 155, 158, 159, 160, 161, 162, 165, 167, 168, 172, 173, 176, 177
clinical manifestations in adults, 7
clinical manifestations in children, 6
clinical presentation, 7, 35, 49, 72
clinical symptoms, 21, 26, 66, 81, 182
clozapine, 82, 84, 137
CNS, 83, 85, 123, 128, 158
cognition, 114, 115, 119, 135
cognitive impairment, 88, 101, 114, 115, 141, 147, 152
collagen, 44, 45, 47
colonization, 12, 15, 16
color, 133, 139, 157
complications, 14, 17, 59, 85, 107, 114, 115, 116, 136, 171, 180, 182
computed tomography, 10, 18, 60
consensus, 16, 18, 43, 52, 55, 76, 81, 160, 161
controversial, 18, 19, 29
correlation(s), 5, 12, 27, 35, 39, 49, 51, 60
cost, 21, 35, 42
cough, 6, 7, 8, 11, 14, 16, 21, 25, 49, 55
covering, vii, viii, 70
culture, 16, 18, 20, 28, 44, 45, 46, 47, 64, 144
cystic fibrosis, 6, 14, 15, 16, 21, 26, 50, 56, 58, 60, 62

D

daily living, 107
deep brain stimulation, 96, 98, 107, 113, 134, 147, 152
defects, 4, 6, 20, 23, 28, 29, 31, 32, 33, 34, 37, 39, 42, 45, 48, 50, 53, 54, 56, 61, 63, 64, 181, 182
deficiency, 32, 33, 118, 141, 169
deficit, 13, 30, 99, 142
dementia, 115, 163, 167
depression, 83, 88, 97, 133, 138, 173
diabetes, 75, 93, 116
diagnosis, 5, 6, 12, 13, 17, 18, 20, 21, 24, 25, 26, 28, 29, 31, 34, 35, 38, 39, 40, 42, 43, 44, 46, 47, 48, 50, 51, 52, 54, 55, 60, 61, 62, 63, 64, 65, 66, 67, 70, 71, 87, 133, 140, 143, 155, 159, 160, 161, 167, 177, 181, 182
diagnostics, 21, 24, 51, 67, 144
disability, 34, 79, 87, 147, 151
disease history, 4
diseases, vii, 2, 5, 7, 14, 20, 21, 26, 35, 47, 49, 52, 105, 106, 143, 168, 172
disorder, viii, 65, 69, 70, 71, 82, 87, 113, 117, 118, 142, 144, 146, 148, 151, 153, 175, 180, 181, 182
distress, 6, 35, 48, 55, 114
DNA, 16, 38, 168
dopamine, 73, 88, 95, 98, 100, 101, 104, 109, 112
dopaminergic, 70, 76, 78, 106, 107, 110, 119, 142
dosage, 73, 82, 84, 108
drainage, 19, 51, 183
drugs, viii, 4, 68, 69, 70, 76, 78, 81, 82, 84, 85, 87, 97, 99, 104, 105, 107, 112, 144, 180
dyskinesia, v, vii, viii, 4, 20, 25, 27, 28, 30, 46, 47, 54, 64, 69, 71, 72, 75, 86, 87, 88, 89, 90, 91, 93, 94, 96, 97, 99, 100, 101,

103, 104, 105, 106, 107, 108, 109, 110, 111, 112, 113, 117, 118, 119, 120, 121, 124, 125, 126, 127, 128, 129, 130, 133, 134, 138, 141, 145, 148, 152, 159, 160, 162, 170, 177, 179, 182, 183
dystonia, viii, 71, 74, 75, 86, 95, 96, 99, 101, 103, 104, 105, 113, 114, 117, 118, 119, 132, 133, 134, 140, 148, 153, 160, 162, 164, 180

E

edema, 148, 153, 168
editors, 133, 155, 165, 167, 176
effusion, 6, 51, 60
electron, 21, 22, 23, 24, 28, 29, 31, 32, 63, 64
electron microscopy, 21, 22, 23, 24, 32, 63, 64
endoscopy, 9, 10, 144
England, 53, 55, 56, 57, 64
ENT clinical manifestations, 8
ENT treatment, 17
enzyme(s), 16, 81, 107, 166
epidemiology, vii, viii, 70, 92, 168
epilepsy, 106, 118, 134
epithelial cells, 3, 39, 44, 67, 68
epithelium, 26, 27, 44, 50, 64
ERS, 20, 21, 22, 24, 43, 58, 61, 183
essential tremor, 134, 147, 151, 163
etiology, vii, viii, 70, 117, 160, 161
evidence, ix, 15, 18, 72, 73, 74, 81, 82, 85, 86, 87, 92, 104, 106, 111, 142, 180, 182
evolution, 3, 7, 9, 18, 49, 51, 164, 165, 166
exercise, vii, ix, 15, 18, 103, 104, 105, 106, 107, 109, 110, 113, 115, 116, 118, 119, 183
exposure, 25, 45, 60, 72, 73, 76, 77, 87, 88, 174, 180

F

false positive, 29, 31, 43, 50
families, 31, 34, 89, 100
fertility, vii, 2, 12, 19, 48, 49
fertility problems, 12, 48
fibrosis, 16, 60, 145, 172
fluctuations, 8, 71, 107
fluid, 3, 18, 144
formation, 44, 65, 80, 166, 182
free radicals, 80, 85, 93

G

GABA, 77, 78, 79, 84, 85, 94, 100
gait, 108, 113, 114, 115, 141, 148, 153, 180
gene therapy, 19, 47, 52, 68, 183
gene therapy in PCD, 19, 47
general measures, 14, 81, 82
genes, viii, 2, 6, 7, 12, 13, 19, 23, 31, 32, 33, 34, 35, 37, 38, 39, 40, 42, 50, 79, 91, 101, 118, 182
genetic analysis in PCD, 35
genetic disease, vii, viii, 2
genetic mutations, 39, 50, 51
genetic predisposition, 79, 180
genetic testing, viii, 2, 24, 51
genetics, vii, viii, 2, 21, 24, 27, 31, 43, 50, 51, 61, 65, 91, 101, 125, 165, 166, 167, 168
genomics, 55, 165, 166
genotype, 7, 54, 96
genotype-phenotype correlation, 35
globus, 77, 109, 149, 154
growth, 7, 44, 45, 49
guidelines, 14, 16, 17, 18, 21, 24, 25, 26, 39, 43, 52, 61, 86, 87, 182

H

health, 5, 14, 15, 48, 49, 50, 99, 157, 172
hearing loss, 8, 17, 19, 49, 51, 168
hemorrhage, 149, 153, 168
high-speed video microscopy, 22, 26
history, 50, 95, 140, 143, 144, 172
human, 35, 38, 47, 53, 59, 68, 76, 99, 157, 158, 164, 165, 173
hydrocephalus, 6, 14, 35, 168
hypoplasia, 10, 13, 49
hypothesis, 76, 80, 81, 100

I

iatrogenic, 88, 105, 180
IDA, 23, 29, 31, 38, 40
idiopathic, 9, 59, 99, 118, 163, 164
image(s), 27, 28, 41, 158, 166
immunofluorescence, viii, 2, 21, 24, 32, 38, 41, 42, 45, 47, 50, 52, 66, 67
impairments, 113, 115, 119
in vitro, 19, 45, 47, 61, 110
incidence, 29, 72, 89, 93, 94, 114, 180, 182
individuals, 6, 44, 91, 104
infarction, 149, 153, 168
infection, 11, 12, 16, 18, 25, 27, 30, 49, 57, 62
infertility, 12, 35, 49, 56
inheritance, viii, 2, 31
inhibition, 77, 83, 93
injury/injuries, 110, 114, 169
intervention, 115, 116, 180
issues, vii, 2, 63, 114, 136, 140, 171, 177

L

L-3,4-dihydroxyphenylalanine (L-DOPA), 106, 107, 108, 109, 110, 111, 121, 124, 127

laterality, 6, 13, 31, 48, 56
L-DOPA-induced dyskinesia (LIDs), ix, 103, 106, 108, 109, 110, 118, 119, 121, 124, 127
lead, 4, 6, 20, 29, 31, 43, 77, 79, 80, 82, 89, 148, 152
legs, 117, 132, 164
lesions, 49, 110, 169
levodopa-induced dyskinesia, ix, 103, 104, 162
light, 29, 104, 132
longitudinal study, 7, 55, 56, 57
lower respiratory tract infection, 7, 14, 182
lung disease, 14, 18, 20, 21, 57, 58, 60, 172
lung function, 7, 11, 15, 16, 17, 21, 35, 49, 51, 58

M

majority, viii, 2, 71, 86, 116, 146, 151
management, 14, 16, 18, 19, 21, 51, 53, 54, 58, 60, 63, 92, 95, 134, 140, 144, 148, 153, 155, 180, 181, 182
manganese, 79, 81, 101
measurement, 25, 26, 27, 61
media, 8, 49, 51
medical, 17, 19, 24, 51, 86, 104, 115
medication, 71, 72, 75, 83, 87, 89, 101, 104, 105, 115, 137, 147, 152, 180
medicine, 143, 157, 180
mental illness, viii, 70, 88, 89, 113, 138, 176
meta-analysis, 7, 55, 58, 72, 91, 97, 99
methodology, 39, 40, 45
mice, 107, 109, 110, 111
microscope, 27, 28, 29
microscopy, 29, 32, 33, 38, 156
mitochondrial DNA, 170
models, 14, 19, 76, 106, 107, 115, 119, 134, 166, 173
molecules, viii, 69, 80, 83
mortality, 105, 114, 115

movement disorders, 90, 94, 95, 97, 100, 104, 105, 111, 114, 130, 139, 140, 160, 161, 162, 163, 164, 177, 179
mucosa, 26, 28, 44, 68
mucus, 15, 27, 43, 44, 182
muscles, 70, 86, 168
mutant, 41, 67, 165
mutation(s), viii, 2, 6, 7, 11, 20, 23, 27, 31, 32, 33, 35, 38, 39, 40, 42, 56, 65, 66, 67, 118, 140, 141, 147, 152, 165, 170
myoclonus, 104, 114, 134, 140, 142, 164, 180

N

neurodegeneration, 109, 112, 163
neuroleptics, viii, 69, 70, 90, 99, 113
neurons, 107, 110, 112
neurotransmitter, 76, 78, 80, 81, 95, 106
nitric oxide, 21, 22, 23, 24, 25, 35, 50, 61, 62
nucleus/nuclei, 41, 86, 96, 149, 153

O

organ(s), vii, 2, 3, 13, 48, 97, 145
other clinical manifestations, 13
otitis media, 6, 7, 8, 17, 19, 49, 51, 60
oxygen, 6, 17, 116, 144

P

pain, 70, 134, 148, 152, 168
parkinsonism, 74, 77, 83, 84, 88, 111, 132, 140, 141, 163
Parkinson's disease (PD), 104, 106, 107, 108, 111, 119, 141, 146, 151
paroxysmal dyskinesias (PxDs), 105, 117, 119, 170
pathogenesis, 53, 76, 180

pathology, 14, 29, 75, 180
pathophysiology, 63, 96, 112, 135, 144, 160, 161, 180, 181
pathway(s), 11, 24, 49, 50, 76
PCD genes classification, 31
penetrance, 100, 146, 151
PET, 77, 98, 123, 127, 134, 159
pH, 27, 29, 43
phenomenology, 100, 114, 117, 160, 161
phenotype(s), 7, 12, 32, 35, 46, 47, 54, 57, 58, 65, 68, 118, 141, 182
physical activity, vii, ix, 103, 106, 116, 119
physical exercise, 15, 18, 104, 106, 107, 110, 115, 118, 119, 183
physiopathology, 76, 80, 88, 160, 162
placebo, 83, 85, 90, 94, 96, 97, 98, 101
plasma levels, 85, 98, 107
plasticity, 76, 80, 81
polymorphism, 79, 94, 95, 99
polyps, 9, 18, 145
population, 5, 12, 20, 42, 57, 71, 105, 114, 115, 166
prevention, 70, 81, 86, 87, 168, 180, 181, 183
preventive approach, viii, 70, 89
primary ciliary dyskinesia, v, vii, 1, 2, 4, 5, 20, 21, 27, 28, 36, 41, 48, 52, 53, 54, 55, 56, 57, 58, 59, 60, 61, 62, 63, 64, 65, 66, 67, 68, 156, 165, 172, 181, 182
primary ciliary dyskinesia in rare diseases context, 5
probability, 72, 74, 75
professionals, 48, 51, 140
prognosis, 12, 48, 88, 144, 181
propranolol, 90, 97, 98
proteins, viii, 2, 31, 32, 33, 34, 38, 39, 40, 42, 50, 182
Pseudomonas aeruginosa, 7, 10, 12, 59
psychosis, 88, 89, 93, 96, 100
pulmonary clinical manifestations, 11
pulmonary management, 15

Q

quality of life, 7, 15, 16, 38, 48, 49, 58, 87, 107, 146, 151
quetiapine, 82, 84, 93

R

radiation, 18, 25, 60, 169
reactions, 74, 89, 97, 108
receptor(s), 70, 76, 77, 78, 79, 80, 82, 84, 95, 98, 99, 100, 101107,, 112
recommendations, 14, 21, 55, 60, 87, 182
rehabilitation, ix, 103, 108, 113, 114, 171
relevance, 63, 110, 136
remission, 71, 72, 86
researchers, 19, 156, 158
resolution, 18, 55, 60, 136
response, ix, 8, 17, 96, 100, 104, 113
rhinitis, 6, 7, 8, 48
rhinorrhea, 8, 11, 49
risk(s), viii, 15, 17, 70, 71, 72, 73, 74, 75, 76, 78, 79, 82, 84, 86, 87, 89, 90, 91, 92, 93, 94, 97, 98, 99, 105, 114, 115, 116, 147, 151
risk factors, 72, 94, 98, 99, 105

S

schizophrenia, ix, 71, 79, 87, 88, 92, 94, 97, 98, 99, 100, 101, 103, 105, 115, 116, 132, 137, 175, 179, 183
screening tests, 25, 182
second generation, 91, 116, 184
sensitivity, 26, 28, 79
serotonin, 79, 98, 99
sex, 7, 73, 138, 166
showing, 31, 32, 33, 70, 108
side effects, 83, 84, 85, 86, 87, 106, 111, 183
signs, 106, 141, 174
sinuses, 10, 11, 49
sinusitis, 4, 6, 8, 18, 26
situs inversus, vii, 2, 4, 5, 6, 7, 11, 13, 30, 31, 53, 54, 182
smoking, 14, 92, 116, 117
Spain, 1, 2, 5, 69
specificities for adult management, 18
speech, 51, 88, 113, 141
sperm, 3, 19, 181
stability, 71, 86, 113
state(s), 51, 55, 62, 77, 78, 134
stimulation, 78, 133, 134, 135, 136, 146, 148, 150, 153, 155, 168, 174
stress, 71, 92, 106
striatum, 77, 78, 107, 109, 110, 111, 119
structure, viii, 2, 3, 28, 29, 30, 32, 33, 48, 57
suspensions, 44, 45, 47
symptoms, vii, 2, 4, 5, 6, 7, 18, 21, 34, 40, 58, 71, 74, 80, 82, 83, 84, 88, 89, 93, 97, 99, 104, 105, 106, 107, 110, 119, 149, 153, 167, 183
synaptic plasticity, 80, 100, 112
syndrome, 4, 11, 13, 26, 30, 34, 37, 48, 53, 54, 57, 58, 59, 60, 61, 64, 87, 88, 95, 96, 100, 105, 115, 134, 140, 145, 163, 164, 168, 177
synthesis, 77, 81, 89, 94, 107, 112

T

tardive dyskinesia (TD), vii, viii, ix, 69, 70, 71, 72, 73, 74, 75, 76, 77, 78, 79, 80, 81, 82, 83, 84, 85, 86, 87, 88, 89, 90, 91, 92, 93, 94, 95, 96, 97, 98, 99, 100, 101, 103, 104, 105, 106, 111, 112, 113, 114, 115, 116, 119, 132, 133, 162, 163, 174, 176, 183
tardive dyskinesia and paroxysmal dyskinesia, 104
target, 40, 42, 107, 149, 154

Task Force, 5, 124, 183
techniques, 15, 25, 38, 62, 133, 135, 147, 151, 158, 177
technology/technologies, 35, 76, 112
TEM, viii, 2, 22, 23, 28, 30, 31, 39, 40, 42, 43, 45, 46, 47, 50, 51
temperature, 27, 39, 43
testing, 18, 23, 24, 67, 115, 168
thalamus, 147, 149, 151, 154
therapeutics, 132, 144, 172
therapy, 6, 17, 18, 47, 52, 59, 61, 93, 96, 101, 106, 107, 135, 144, 145
tics, 104, 114, 140, 141, 160, 162, 163, 180
tissue, 3, 43, 44, 134
training, 108, 110, 115, 140
transmission, 19, 32, 49, 64, 80, 146, 151
transmission electron microscopy, viii, 2, 28, 32, 64
transplant, 17, 107, 142
transport, 4, 12, 30, 31, 49, 50, 53, 96, 113
treatment, viii, 2, 7, 8, 11, 14, 16, 17, 18, 19, 30, 38, 48, 49, 50, 51, 52, 55, 59, 60, 70, 74, 79, 80, 81, 82, 83, 84, 85, 86, 87, 89, 90, 92, 93, 94, 95, 96, 97, 98, 100, 101, 106, 107, 108, 110, 111, 113, 118, 120, 122, 123, 124, 125, 126, 127, 130, 133, 134, 140, 143, 144, 146, 150, 151, 154, 155, 160, 161, 168, 179, 180, 181, 182, 183
tremor, 114, 134, 140, 141, 146, 147, 151, 163, 170, 180
trial, 16, 58, 59, 90, 92, 93, 94, 101, 115

U

ultrastructure, viii, 2, 4, 21, 27, 28, 29, 30, 31, 33, 40, 42, 43, 46, 51, 62, 63, 66
United States, 59, 83, 120, 123, 125, 127, 181
upper respiratory tract, 27, 49, 59

V

Valencia, 1, 2, 69
variations, 79, 81, 90
ventilation, 6, 17, 116
videos, 50, 140, 177
vision, 27, 47, 135, 142, 168

W

walking, ix, 104, 114, 115, 116
withdrawal, 96, 174, 180